PSYCHIATRY - THEORY, APPLICATIONS AND TREATMENTS

INNOVATIONS IN PSYCHIATRY

Psychiatry - Theory, Applications and Treatments

Additional books and e-books in this series can be found on Nova's website under the Series tab.

PSYCHIATRY - THEORY, APPLICATIONS AND TREATMENTS

INNOVATIONS IN PSYCHIATRY

SOUPARNO MITRA
URMI CHAUDHURI
AND
PANAGIOTA KORENIS
EDITORS

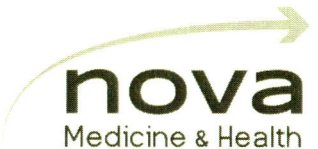

Copyright © 2021 by Nova Science Publishers, Inc.

All rights reserved. No part of this book may be reproduced, stored in a retrieval system or transmitted in any form or by any means: electronic, electrostatic, magnetic, tape, mechanical photocopying, recording or otherwise without the written permission of the Publisher.

We have partnered with Copyright Clearance Center to make it easy for you to obtain permissions to reuse content from this publication. Simply navigate to this publication's page on Nova's website and locate the "Get Permission" button below the title description. This button is linked directly to the title's permission page on copyright.com. Alternatively, you can visit copyright.com and search by title, ISBN, or ISSN.

For further questions about using the service on copyright.com, please contact:
Copyright Clearance Center
Phone: +1-(978) 750-8400   Fax: +1-(978) 750-4470   E-mail: info@copyright.com.

NOTICE TO THE READER

The Publisher has taken reasonable care in the preparation of this book, but makes no expressed or implied warranty of any kind and assumes no responsibility for any errors or omissions. No liability is assumed for incidental or consequential damages in connection with or arising out of information contained in this book. The Publisher shall not be liable for any special, consequential, or exemplary damages resulting, in whole or in part, from the readers' use of, or reliance upon, this material. Any parts of this book based on government reports are so indicated and copyright is claimed for those parts to the extent applicable to compilations of such works.

Independent verification should be sought for any data, advice or recommendations contained in this book. In addition, no responsibility is assumed by the Publisher for any injury and/or damage to persons or property arising from any methods, products, instructions, ideas or otherwise contained in this publication.

This publication is designed to provide accurate and authoritative information with regard to the subject matter covered herein. It is sold with the clear understanding that the Publisher is not engaged in rendering legal or any other professional services. If legal or any other expert assistance is required, the services of a competent person should be sought. FROM A DECLARATION OF PARTICIPANTS JOINTLY ADOPTED BY A COMMITTEE OF THE AMERICAN BAR ASSOCIATION AND A COMMITTEE OF PUBLISHERS.

Additional color graphics may be available in the e-book version of this book.

Library of Congress Cataloging-in-Publication Data

ISBN: 978-1-53619-365-7

Published by Nova Science Publishers, Inc. † New York

Contents

Preface		vii
Acknowledgments		xi
Chapter 1	Technological Cycles in Psychiatry *Urmi Chaudhuri*	1
Chapter 2	Telepsychiatry and Its Use across Subspecialties in Psychiatry *Aditya Sareen and Panagiota Korenis*	11
Chapter 3	Apps for Anxiety *Arun George Prasad*	21
Chapter 4	Journaling Apps *Maria Alejandra Gallo-Ruiz*	33
Chapter 5	c-CBT *Aditya Sareen and Bibiana Susaimanickam*	43
Chapter 6	Apps for Eating Disorders *Ingrid Haza*	59
Chapter 7	PSYCKES and PDMP *Gurtej Singh Gill and Sasidhar Gunturu*	71

Chapter 8	Ecological Momentary Assessment (EMA) *Souparno Mitra*	85
Chapter 9	Apps for Child and Adolescent Mental Health Disorders *Himansh Saxena*	101
Chapter 10	Apps for Attention-Deficit Hyperactivity Disorder (ADHD) *Monika Gashi*	115
Chapter 11	Apps for Substance Use Disorders *Kiran Jose*	127
Chapter 12	Psychological Testing Tools *Khai Tran*	137
Chapter 13	Social Media and Its Impact on Mental Health *Noemi Edwards*	149
Chapter 14	Future Directions *Shalini Dutta and Souparno Mitra*	157

About the Editors   165

Index   167

PREFACE

This book will present the most up to date and concise information related to psychiatric innovations and is especially written for those looking for a quick and easy reference guide. Conveniently formatted to present the most current and up to date concepts and ensure that you are prepared for your psychiatry shelf, PRITE™, psychiatry boards and recertification exams. It will quickly become your go to reference material for psychiatric technological innovations.

Chapter 1 - In this chapter, the authors take a walk down memory lane. The authors review the long history of psychiatric illnesses and assessment modalities. The authors look at times where asylums were the only modality of treatment to today when we have telepsychiatry. The authors also discuss the different cycles of development of technology and how that may play in to the field of psychiatry. This chapter will give a strong starting point to the rest of the chapters discussed in this book.

Chapter 2 - In this chapter, the authors discuss the benefits and uses of Telepsychiatry in a clinical setting. The authors start with the description of Telepsychiatry and explore the benefits of Telepsychiatry as well as potential challenges. The authors then examine the evidence of the use of Telepsychiatry in different subspecialty settings such as Child and Adolescent psychiatry, Geriatric psychiatry, Consultant and liaison psychiatry, Addiction psychiatry and Forensic psychiatry.

Chapter 3 - Anxiety disorders are the most common mental illness in the USA and cause significant morbidity and mortality in the USA. In this chapter the authors shall discuss apps used for anxiety which are commonly available in the Android/iOS market, and compare their efficacy and individual rating.

Chapter 4 - Journals have been used for documents, thoughts and feelings for aeons. With the advent of smartphones, journaling applications have been developed and people have been able to document their thoughts and feelings in real-time. In the authors' chapter, they will discuss the different options of applications that are available for use in journaling and the different kinds of journaling that do exist.

Chapter 5 - Cognitive behavioral therapy (CBT) is an evidence-based treatment modality used to treat depression, anxiety, stress, eating disorders, post-traumatic stress disorder (PTSD) and related mental challenges. CBT actively engages the patient in addressing these issues by learning new ways of thinking, feeling and behaving that promote improved self-care and mental wellness.

With the advent of the internet and mobile devices, increasingly, mental health organizations are offering an online version of this approach called "computerized CBT" or c- CBT. As the demand for mental health services increases, providers are seeking new ways to assist larger population in the most efficient manner. The c-CBT approach directly addresses this need. In this chapter the authors discuss about advantages and limitations of c-CBT and its utilization specifically in treatment of depression, anxiety, insomnia and eating disorders.

Chapter 6 - Mobile apps have significantly evolved since their inception in 1994. This is especially true of mobile apps developed for eating disorders. Whether they aid as an adjunct for therapy or treatment of patients afflicted with eating disorders, these are gaining more traction within the community of providers treating these disorders. Throughout the years different principles have been developed, which have impacted the way patients and providers use said apps. This chapter explores the development of apps, their use, their limitations, and studies available which compare and contrast the pros and cons of apps for eating disorders.

Chapter 7 - This chapter will discuss the importance of Psychiatric Services and Clinical Knowledge Enhancement System (PSYCKES) and Prescription Drug Monitoring Program (PDMP). The authors will start with the Introduction of PSYCKES and PDMP and will discuss sample cases. Later, the authors will discuss the practicality of the magnificent clinical database, its limitations, and future direction for utilizing this database for their patients.

Chapter 8 - In this chapter, the authors discuss the importance of Ecological Momentary Assessment. The authors start with a description of what Ecological Momentary Assessment is and move on to discuss its applications as it relates to clinical work and research as well as the advantages and disadvantages of this methodology. The authors also review papers which have looked into the efficacy of this intervention and discuss the future of this methodology.

Chapter 9 - This chapter has a brief description of the various mental illnesses and the free online resources that are available to administer children. The importance of having free online resources at the disposal of parents or caregivers to administer in the time of uncertainty is of paramount. Having access to free online applications with a push or a click of a button on their cell phone or a computer can help caregivers with children to seek proper care for the child. It is by far one of the most essential tools a caregiver should have in their arsenal when dealing with various mental illnesses that stricken children at various age groups. These online tools can educate and direct a parent, a guardian, a teacher, a babysitter or any adult taking care of a child to seek physician's care if needed.

Chapter 10 - Attention deficit hyperactivity disorder (ADHD) is a chronic mental health condition. It can present with pattern of inattention with or without hyperactivity and or impulsivity, resulting in impairment in functioning. Some of the major functions that are affected especially in childhood are social, emotional, and cognitive development, necessary for shaping a child for adulthood. By the end this chapter you will be able to narrate the history of ADHD, its neurobiology, established treatment and available applications for patient with ADHD and their care givers, presented through a sample case.

Chapter 11 - In this chapter, the authors discuss the role of mobile health apps that facilitate recovery from substance use disorders.

The authors start the chapter by understanding the definition and the diagnostic criteria used for substance use disorders along with some recent epidemiological data. The authors then discuss how mobile apps incorporates pharmacological and behavioral interventions to help patients with substance use disorders.

Benefits and shortcomings of these mobile phone-based health inventions are acknowledged as well and further studies are required to gauge the efficacy and functionality of these apps.

Chapter 12 - With the advancement of technology, as of 2020, the smart phone penetration rate globally is 45.4%. The accessibility of the information highway made it easier to communicate between patient and provider but also allows ease of access to educational information. In this chapter, the authors look at the smart phone applications that would allow screening and evaluation for mental disorder as well as the near future direction that would streamline care for patient and provider.

Chapter 13 - In this chapter, the authors discuss the importance of something that has become ubiquitous with our life: social media. Whether it be Twitter, Instagram, Facebook or TikTok, social media is omnipotent and omnipresent. The authors discuss the impact of social media in our lives, in the mental health of patients and the ways and means that we can overcome the problems that come with social media use.

Chapter 14 - In this chapter the authors discuss the road ahead in the development of new tools and assessments in Psychiatry. The authors discuss the utility of Artificial Intelligence, Face Mapping Softwares, Telepsychiatry and other modalities. Technology is always progressing and improving and the authors' chapter will give insight into some directions that the field of psychiatry can head down.

Acknowledgments

The authors would like to acknowledge Dr Ketki Shah, MD, Chair of the Department of Psychiatry, Bronxcare Health Systems and all the authors on all the chapters for their hard work and perseverance.

We would also like to thank the healthcare workers all over the world who have been on the frontlines fighting this pandemic and have shown their resilience and bravery. A big thank you to you all!

In: Innovations in Psychiatry
Editors: Souparno Mitra et al.
ISBN: 978-1-53619-365-7
© 2021 Nova Science Publishers, Inc.

Chapter 1

TECHNOLOGICAL CYCLES IN PSYCHIATRY

Urmi Chaudhuri, BA (LLB), MHRM*
Isenberg School of Management, Amherst, MA, US

ABSTRACT

In this chapter, we take a walk down memory lane. We review the long history of psychiatric illnesses and assessment modalities. We look at times where asylums were the only modality of treatment to today when we have telepsychiatry. We also discuss the different cycles of development of technology and how that may play in to the field of psychiatry. This chapter will give a strong starting point to the rest of the chapters discussed in this book.

HISTORY OF PSYCHIATRY

In ancient times, people with psychiatric illnesses were labelled witches, imprisoned, feared to be possessed or driven to the wilderness. In the time of Hippocrates or Socrates, mental illness was often assumed to be

---

* Corresponding Author's Email: urmi.chaudhuri@gmail.com.

a spiritual phenomenon. Socrates assumed it to be hysteria, caused by "the womb" wandering around the body causing problems. The treatment he proposed was to have babies in order to keep the womb in the right place.

History shows us that the first asylums came into being in the 8th Century. Britain established their first asylum system in 1300s. Until the 17th century, the concept of humors was thought to be the cause of mental illness and treatment included: warm, cold, purging, bloodletting, diet, activity, rest and exercise etc. In Persia, the first mental hospitals were established where treatment included bath, drugs, music, activity and counselling.

Mental asylums became the main method of containing mental illness. People were institutionalized, kept in extremely unhygienic and poor conditions, often chained and subjected to gross negligence. This has been the subject of many historical documentaries and the cause of many reservations in order to get psychiatric treatments.

Dorothea Dix in the 1800s was a major proponent of mental health advocacy. Her work was instrumental in the expansion of 32 psychiatric hospitals in US, Canada and Europe. Emil Kraeplin was the first person to differentiate between schizophrenia and mania. Eugene Beuler was the first person to coin the term Schizophrenia. Freud contributed by establishing the psychoanalytical model of treatment.

In 1954, the first psychiatric medication *chlorpromazine* was discovered, and this revolutionized mental health care. In the 1900s, James Watts and Walker started the controversial method of Lobotomy, which affected Rosemary Kennedy (John F. Kennedy's sister), leaving her incapacitated. Soon, the Community Mental Health Act was passed in 1963 leading to de-institutionalization. The Diagnostic and Statistical Manual 1st Edition came out in 1952 and American Psychiatric Association was also founded in the 1900s.

We have come a long way in the field of psychiatry: from being a field fraught with controversies to now becoming one of the most important health care fields that is receiving attention. The importance of psychosocial measures have been established including wraparound services such as Assisted Outpatient Treatment, Assertive Community

Treatment, Case Managers and Supervised Residences. These services aim at restoring individuals with mental health illnesses to being able to function in society.

TECHNOLOGICAL LIFE CYCLES

Technological Life Cycles (TLC) is a very well-studied concept in the development of technologies. This described the commercial gain of a product through the research and development phase and the return during its "vital life." The technology underlying the product may be quite different to the process of creating and managing its product. All forms of technology, whether it be cellphones, tablets, computers, all go through the following stages:

1. Innovation Phase
2. Syndication Phase
3. Diffusion Phase
4. Substitution Phase.

Innovation Phase

This is the phase that represents the birth of a product, material or process as a result of research and development (R&D) activities. In R&D labs, new ideas are developed depending on market surveys and the knowledge of current needs. Resources are allocated depending on the change element and the time taken in this phase varies dependent of these factors.

Syndication Phase

This phase is hallmarked by the demonstration, advertising and commercialization of the product. Many products do not even make it to this stage and are kept in the R&D labs. Commercialization of these products depends on technical, non-technical and economic factors.

Diffusion Phase

In this phase this product makes inroads into the market as the consumers accept the innovation and it receives widespread acclaim. However, supply and demand plays a huge role in the rate of diffusion.

Substitution Phase

The last stage is when the technology declines in use. Its functionality is extended and eventually replaced by another technology, being influenced by many technical and non-technical factors.

These cycles can be seen with most technologies. Take for example the case of computers. Computers went from being large circuits connected by wires occupying a whole room to desktop computers which gradually became more and more user friendly and improved in functionality. Dominant models such as the Macbook from Apple and others developed and currently we are in a world of touchscreen laptops.

TECHNOLOGICAL ADVANCES IN PSYCHIATRY

The technological advances in psychiatry have been immense. From being a field where evaluation was based purely on observation and treatments were initially limited to only therapy to now where there is wide utilization of objective scales, imaging, long acting medications, gene testing for drug efficacy, identification of genotypes and most importantly, telepsychiatry, the field has witnessed great technological advancements.

Aaron Beck is known for his development of the Depression and Anxiety Inventory which has great construct validity and reliability.

Hamilton Depression Scale was developed in 1960. It was indeed in the second half of the 20th century that these scales became more popular and the number of scales increased.

The beginning of neuropsychiatry is attributed to the 19th century scientists from France and Germany including Georget, Bayle and Griesinger who hypothesized that mental illnesses have an organic basis and mental disorders were similar to dementia. Their work influenced many neuropsychiatrists such as Meyer, Meynert, Oppenheim, Charcot, Korsakoff, Freud, Bleuler and Kraeplin among others. This investigation into neurological basis of mental illnesses was lost in the beginning of the 20th century due to the growing popularity of the psychodynamic model. Migration of scientists to the United States in the 1900s increased the interest in translational research. With the American Association of Neurology and the American Board of Psychiatry being united into the American Board of Psychiatry and Neurology in 1965, there was a great increase in the research on the neurological basis of mental illness. Today, functional and structural changes in the brain have been identified for Schizophrenia, Obsessive Compulsive Disorders, Major Depression and Bipolar Disorders. This research is still in its early stages and there is still much that is left to be discovered.

Gene testing for antidepressant efficacy was developed using the cytochrome p450 genotyping. Long acting injections were developed beginning in the 1960s, with Fluphenazine decanoate coming into the market in 1968 and the second generation antipsychotics making it into the market between 2003-2013.

The biggest technological advancement in psychiatry has been in the field of Telepsychiatry. The use of videoconferencing dates back to the 1950s when the Nebraska Psychiatric Institute in 1959 used it to provide group therapy and consultation services in the Nebraska State Hospital. In 1969, Massachusetts General Hospital consulted with Logan international Airport's Health Clinic. By the last decade of the 20th century, it had spread to multiple areas of the world and became popular as it eliminated geographical barriers to care. In the 2000s, research on telepsychiatry showed it to be as efficacious as un person care, being equivalent in diagnostic accuracy and treatment. Multiple softwares have been developed to use telepsychiatry which are HIPAA Compliant and regulations have been established by the governing bodies for provision of telepsychiatry. This form of care has become especially important during the COVID-19 pandemic in 2020 when people were unable to visit the clinics or their substance use programs, and more and more psychiatrists are becoming proficient in this field.

LITERATURE REVIEW

Technological Innovations in Mental Healthcare: Harnessing the Digital Revolution (Hollis et al., 2015)

The paper discusses the different elements of technological innovations available in mental health care. They describe that the internet has become an extremely potent too in today's day and age. The advent of tablet PCs and the internet has paved the way for the use of E-Health and m-Health. These terms describe the delivery of healthcare via electronic means using the internet using a variety of devices.

These technologies can improve access to healthcare and treatment adherence by allowing services to be delivered flexibly and tailored to individual needs. Sensor technologies, online psychological therapy and remote video consultations as well as mobile and apps present opportunities to engage and empower patients and create novel approaches.

This paper goes on to talk of the deficits in access to mental healthcare in the National Health Service (NHS) in U. K. The Government developed a strategy "no health without mental health" which recommends increased use of information and communication technology.

E-Health represents a cultural change in healthcare that empowers patients by offering greater choice and control like availability of psychological interventions 24 x 7. Xenzone, Psychology Online and Big White Wall are resources available in NHS.

The paper talks of mental health apps and their use in administering scales, using measures through sensors such as accelerometers, gyroscopes, microphones and cameras. Technological innovations have the potential; of bringing more objectivity and reliability to the diagnostic process.

They also talk of affective computing which is a branch of science that aim to develop automated assessment of a person's mood by analysis of facial expressions. ICT can address issues such as isolation in young people with the use of social media platforms. NHS has established a m Health app library which has as on 2015, 23 apps. However, regulation is difficult and governing bodies are having a tough time keeping up with the speed of development. Other apps they mention include ClinTouch, My Journey, Buddy App and Well Happy.

These developments pose a "big data challenges" for menta health. The use of Electronic Medical Records connected devices as well as e-prescribing has led to the production of a large amount of data that can be of use to researchers.

The paper summarizes that technology is one of the ways forward to bridge the gaps in access to care. However, these methods are subjected to challenges such as ensuring that the patients and their needs remain at the center of development, rapidly increasing the evidence base of these methods and ensuring ways to increase data sharing that does not threaten patient privacy.

Digital Technologies in Psychiatry: Present and Future (Hirschtritt, 2018)

This paper talks of the roads ahead in technological innovations. There are 2.4 billion smartphones in circulation and over two trillion searches annually on Google. The paper asks will clinics be replaced by teleclinicians? Will artificial intelligence (AI) bots replace psychiatrists?

This paper too talks of how digital innovations such as AI, Virtual Reality and Machine Learning can improve various elements such as objective and standardized assessments with continuous ecological measurements of emotion, cognition and behavior. The second problem that technology would address is the access to healthcare in terms of finding resources to start care and also avoid delays in initiation. For example, for first episode psychosis in community clinics, the wait time is 74 weeks. Mental health care is also fragmented, with multiple providers, different treatments and perspectives making the navigation of the system a maze. These systems may lack continuity of care making the availability of technology a boon. The final problem that they address is attitudinal barriers or stigma that limit adherence to care. They hope that the availability of these tools enable access to care and bring about an attitudinal change.

They talk of digital phenotyping as the new form of assessment. This utilizes sensor data such as activity and geolocation, human computer interaction and sleep. Digital innovations may improve mental health treatment via telepsychiatry and provision of evidence-based therapies online.

Three prominent trends that are showing promise include use of interventions for patients with serious mental illness. This includes apps for peer support, treatment adherence and cognitive remediation. The second area they speak of is the potential for combining digital and traditional approaches. FDA has approved the use of reset (an app for digital CBT) to be used as a part of comprehensive care plans in this hybrid model. The third trend is the use of chatbots with sophisticated AI. A study found that the use of a fully automated conversational agent reinforced CBT techniques in a text message format and enabled greater decrease in depressive symptoms. Video games are also being used to train attention and executive function. VR technology is being explored for treating conditions such as PTSD and phobias.

In challenges, they speak of the challenges we have discussed, however, they add to it by describing how this can actually widen the gaps in access on the basis of who can access care and who cannot. Current innovations are currently dedicated for adults. Future directions may be to expand these to children and adolescents. Academies need to look at industry models on how to make devices attractive and useful to customers.

Conclusion

In conclusion, the digital age is upon us. We have progressed immensely from the times of asylums and exorcism to the use of smartphones for provision of mental health care.

As with the computer industry, the digital innovations may be a major factor to bring in a new wave in psychiatry. From reducing stigma, to increasing access to care, to ensuring more objective and accurate assessments, the scope for innovations is endless. We, as psychiatrists and researchers, need to educate ourselves and innovate to improve patient care and the provision of care.

In the following chapters we will discuss some of the innovations that exist in the realm of technological innovations in psychiatry. We will conclude with a one-chapter resource summary of our book and some glimpses for the future.

References

[1] Hirschtritt, M. E., and Insel, T. R. (2018). Digital Technologies in Psychiatry: Present and Future. *Focus* (American Psychiatric Publishing), 16(3), 251-258. https://doi.org/10.1176/appi.focus.20180001.

[2] Hollis, C., Morriss, R., Martin, J., Amani, S., Cotton, R., Denis, M., and Lewis, S. (2015). Technological innovations in mental healthcare: harnessing the digital revolution. *The British journal of psychiatry: the journal of mental science,* 206(4), 263-265. https://doi.org/10.1192/bjp.bp.113.142612.

[3] Bayus, B. (1998). An Analysis of Product Lifetimes in a Technologically Dynamic Industry. *Management Science,* 44(6), pp. 763-775.
[4] *Wikipedia.* (2020). Technological life cycles.

Chapter 2

TELEPSYCHIATRY AND ITS USE ACROSS SUBSPECIALTIES IN PSYCHIATRY

Aditya Sareen[1], MD and Panagiota Korenis[1,2,*], MD
[1]BronxCare Health System Department of Psychiatry,
Icahn School of Medicine, New York, NY, US
[2]Albert Einstein College of Medicine, Bronx, NY, US

ABSTRACT

In this chapter, we discuss the benefits and uses of Telepsychiatry in a clinical setting. We start with the description of Telepsychiatry and explore the benefits of Telepsychiatry as well as potential challenges. We then examine the evidence of the use of Telepsychiatry in different subspecialty settings such as Child and Adolescent psychiatry, Geriatric psychiatry, Consultant and liaison psychiatry, Addiction psychiatry and Forensic psychiatry.

---

[*] Corresponding Author's Email: PKorenis@bronxcare.org.

TELEPSYCHIATRY USE AND IMPLICATIONS

Telemedicine is known as the process of providing health care from a distance with the use of technology, often using videoconferencing. Telepsychiatry, is a subset of telemedicine and is focused on providing a range of services including psychiatric evaluations, patient education, therapy (individual therapy, group therapy, family therapy), and psychopharmacological management.

Telepsychiatry may involve the direct interaction between a psychiatrist and the patient. It also affords psychiatrists the opportunity to support primary care providers with mental health care consultation and collaboration. Mental health care can be provided in a live, interactive manner and can also involve recording medical information (images, videos, etc.) and sending this out to a distant site for later review.

Telepsychiatry has a number of benefits and helps create accessible, convenient and affordable mental health services. It can benefit patients in a number of ways including: improving access to mental health care in rural areas where there might be limited opportunities; integration of behavioral health and primary care; reduction of unnecessary emergency room visits; decrease delays in care; improve continuity of care and follow-up; reduce the time needed to commute and other transportation barriers.

Table 1. Benefits of telepsychiatry

Benefits of Telepsychiatry
Patients avoid traveling to the clinic
Clinicians can see patient's home environment
Avoids patient frustration with waiting in a busy wait room
Can increase compliance with appointments
Prevents unnecessary exposure for routine medical appointments for vulnerable patients
Provides clues about social determinants that could influence a patient's physical and emotional health

Table 2. Strategies to convey empathy during telepsychiatry sessions

Tip	Think	Do
Be "present"	What should I do to be ready for the session	Optimize the space to ensure connection (video/audio quality)
	How am I feeling?	Pause, breathe, minimize distractions
	Who is my patient	Invest time in introducing yourself to your patient and hearing them introduce themselves
Identify needs	What do they expect from the clinician	Ask clear and open-ended questions first to elicit patient's needs upfront
		Allow time during the session for the patient to ask you questions so you can understand their concerns
Listen	What are they saying in both content and emotion?	Feelings, concerns, worries Manner in which they are speaking - tone of voice
Respond with empathy	What did I hear, in content and emotion?	Summarize the content "just to summarize, you are stating that you are concerned about your inability to sleep because it is making it hard to function at work." Reflect on what they are saying egs. They tell you about the death of a loved one, rather than "I'm sorry," try "It sounds like it has been a difficult time for you" Name the emotion egs. Patient talks about not being able to pick up prescriptions on time you say "It sounds like this situation really frustrated or upset you"
Share information	Be clear and concise	Distribute information in small amounts
	How can I check understanding	Ask questions, invite the patient to summarize their understanding

Telepsychiatry allows psychiatrists to treat more patients in distant locations. This has served as a critical benefit to providing access of care to those in rural areas where it is difficult to recruit psychiatrists.

TELEPSYCHIATRY CHALLENGES

Despite the benefit of increasing access, not being in the same room as the patient may create enhanced feelings of the need to ensure safety, security and privacy for many patients. Additionally, it may create a space where the patient feels a lack of engagement due to the inability to engage in the usual nonverbal social behaviors. The use of technology and issues with video and sound quality may lead to a sense of disconnect and distraction.

EVIDENCE FOR THE USE OF TELEPSYCHIATRY

There is substantial evidence of the effectiveness and evidence-based use of telepsychiatry. Research has found satisfaction to be high among patients, psychiatrists and other professionals [1]. In terms of research outcomes, studies show that telepsychiatry is equivalent to in-person care in diagnostic accuracy, treatment effectiveness, quality of care and patient satisfaction [2].

Research has also found that overall experiences among all age groups has been positive. There is evidence for children, adolescents and adults regarding assessment and treatment (medication and therapy). There have also been subtypes of patients for which telemedicine may be preferable to in-person care, for example people with autism or severe anxiety disorders and patients with physical limitations may find the remote treatment particularly beneficial.

Telepsychiatry has been found especially effective with respect to the treatment of depression, ADHD and PTSD, depression, and ADHD.

Telepsychiatry is helping bring more timely psychiatric care to emergency rooms. An estimated one in eight emergency room visits involves a patient who presents with a mental health and/or substance use condition [3]. Across the United States, many emergency rooms are not equipped to manage patients with serious mental health issues and do not have ready access to psychiatrists or other mental health clinicians on staff to assess and treat mental health conditions.

TELEPSYCHIATRY IN CHILD AND ADOLESCENT PSYCHIATRY

There are a limited number of child and adolescent psychiatrists to provide care to children and adolescents who are experiencing mental health related concerns. This has created a gap in care that is dire for this particular patient population. Tele psychiatry has emerged as an important technological advancement to bridge the gap between the patients and the providers. This also addresses the concerns of parent concerns about missing work and the children concerns about missing school. There have been some concern whether if the efficacy of Telepsychiatry can be compared to the in-person setting. Hyler et al. In 2005 conducted a study involving 25 patients age 4-16 and compared the efficacy of Telepsychiatry to that of in-person interviews [5]. They found that for 96% of patients the diagnosis and treatment recommendations were the same. Though the psychiatrist did report that it may not be adequate in evaluation of teenage depression and for difficult teenagers who refuse to cooperate.

However, preschool evaluations can have their own distinct challenges. One may require further assistance at a distant site which can be achieved by a parent or a guardian. It is also important to evaluate the satisfaction of children and adolescents utilizing such a service. Myers et al. in 2008 evaluated the utilization and efficacy of a telemedicine service and found that parents endorsed high satisfaction with their school-aged children's care and lower satisfaction with their adolescents' care which could be because adolescents require a larger range of services than offered by the tele psychiatry service [6]. There service was predominantly utilized for diagnosis and medication management. Telepsychiatry thus helps bridge the gap between families who would have not accessed care due to the stigma, the lack of faith in the facility's services, or the inability to obtain the psychiatric services they needed.

TELEPSYCHIATRY IN GERIATRIC SERVICES

With the increase in numbers of individuals above age of 65 in the united states and elsewhere there has been a growing demand for their health care needs. These individuals have chronic health conditions and need specialized medical and mental health care. The number of geriatric mental health providers are inadequate to meet the needs of such a population. This gap can be addressed by Tele-psychiatry. The Medicare program provides health care for majority of patients in the United States. However Medicare also limits the types of Tele-psychiatric reimbursements which results in a potential barrier to its use for geriatric population. A recent systematic review involving 68 studies found telemedicine useful in geriatric populations in the areas of nursing home consultation, screening and diagnosis of cognitive disorders, management of depression in integrated and collaborative care models, and psychotherapy [7].

Patient satisfaction remains an important indicator to determine the utilization of such services in geriatric populations. Hantke et al. evaluated the patient satisfaction of tele-psychiatry service in 45 community-dwelling older Veterans and found that the majority of participants (90%) reported liking or even preferring geriatric Telepsychiatry, despite the experience being novel for the majority of patients [7]. However, critiques also argue that geriatric patients may have sensory impairments and unique aspects to their psychiatric problems. This can make Telepsychiatry health assessments more challenging. It is not clear what model of Telepsychiatry constitutes the best practice for geriatric psychiatry and further research is required [8].

TELEPSYCHIATRY IN CONSULTATION AND LIAISON SERVICES

Psychiatrists play an important role in multi-disciplinary management of patients in the inpatient medical and surgical setting. The lack of psychiatrists in such settings can results in prolonged length of stay for patients with delirium or patients with co-morbid mental illnesses. Due to the lack of psychiatrists at such sites, Telepsychiatry has come up as an important tool to help meet the demand. Some studies have demonstrated successful collaboration using Telepsychiatry between a public, academic medical center, and an unaffiliated, community hospital [9]. Though there are a wide range of benefits from such services, certain challenges still remain, such as acceptability of such service by patients and the cost. Telepsychiatry is not reimbursed by managed care companies in many states.

TELEPSYCHIATRY IN ADDICTION SERVICES

The United states has an opioid epidemic. The prevalence of this epidemic is on the rise and so is the demand for Medication assisted treatment (MAT) for opioid use disorder. Telepsychiatry is a promising way for the delivery of MAT and expand the access of care. Zheng et al., in 2017 conducted a retrospective chart review to assess the difference between face-to-face and Telepsychiatry buprenorphine Medication-assisted treatment (MAT) programs for the treatment of opioid use disorder. They found no statistical difference in in terms of additional substance use, average time to 30 and 90 days of abstinence, and treatment retention rates between Telepsychiatry and face to face treatment [7]. Thereby suggesting that Telepsychiatry may be equally efficacious in delivery of such treatment programs.

TELEPSYCHIATRY IN FORENSIC AND CORRECTIONAL SERVICES

As per recent data from the US Department of Justice, more than 10% of the population in US prisons suffer from mental illness [8]. Correctional facilities often find it difficult to arrange for mental health treatment for such patients. Telepsychiatry has the potential to overcome these challenges. Forensic Telepsychiatry can also help criminal justice agencies such as courts, prisons, and probation to have access to forensic expertise in a timely and efficient manner [9.

Brodey et al. conducted a study to compare satisfaction in 43 forensic psychiatric patient inmates from the general population of the King County Correctional Facility, a large urban jail in Seattle comparing Telepsychiatry visits to in person visits. They found no significant difference between them [10].

One of the most emerging use of Forensic Telepsychiatry is to meet the demand for forensic evaluations among asylum seekers throughout the United States. Forensic evaluators are vital in documenting the psychological sequelae of human rights abuses and explaining the importance to adjudicators of immigration cases [11]. However such centers are underserved in addition to the increasing number of detention centers in the country. Forensic services are therefore highly needed in such areas. Recently Mount Sinai Human Rights Program (MSHRP) launched its Remote Evaluation Network [12]. The Remote Evaluation Network expands MSHRP's reach to asylum seekers in underserved geographies across the US by conducting pro bono forensic mental health evaluations by Telepsychiatry. The Remote Evaluation Network conducted evaluations of individuals in immigration detention facilities, who generally have little to no access to forensic medical services. Thus Telehealth services offers solution for the national need for evaluations and continues to expand access to forensic mental health evaluations.

REFERENCES

[1] Hyler S. E., Gangure D. P., Batchelder S. T. Can telepsychiatry replace in-person psychiatric assessments? A review and meta-analysis of comparison studies CNS Spectrums 200510403413.7. Hyler S. E., Gangure D. P., Batchelder S. T. Can telepsychiatry replace in-person psychiatric assessments? A review and meta-analysis of comparison studies. *CNS Spectrums* 2005;10:403-413.

[2] Myers K. M., Valentine J. M., & Melzer S. M. (2008). Child and adolescent telepsychiatry: utilization and satisfaction. *Telemedicine and e-Health*, 14(2), 131-137.

[3] Melanie T. Gentry, Maria I. Lapid, Teresa A. Rummans, Geriatric Telepsychiatry: Systematic Review and Policy Considerations, *The American Journal of Geriatric Psychiatry*, Volume 27, Issue 2, 2019, Pages 109-127, ISSN 1064-7481, https://doi.org/10.1016/j.jagp.2018.10.009.

[4] Hantke N., Lajoy M., Gould C. E., Magwene E. M., Sordahl J., Hirst, R., & O'Hara R. (2020). Patient Satisfaction with Geriatric Psychiatry Services via Video Teleconference. *The American Journal of Geriatric Psychiatry: Official Journal of the American Association for Geriatric Psychiatry*, 28(4), 491-494. https://doi-org.eresources.mssm.edu/10.1016/j.jagp.2019.08.020.

[5] Jones B. N., 3rd, & Ruskin P. E. (2001). Telemedicine and geriatric psychiatry: directions for future research and policy. *Journal of Geriatric Psychiatry and Neurology*, 14(2), 59-62. https://doi-org.eresources.mssm.edu/10.1177/089198870101400202.

[6] Kimmel R. J., & Toor R. (2019). Telepsychiatry by a Public, Academic Medical Center for Inpatient Consults at an Unaffiliated, Community Hospital. *Psychosomatics*, 60(5), 468-473. https://doi.org/10.1016/j.psym.2018.12.004.

[7] Zheng W., Nickasch M., Lander L., Wen S., Xiao M., Marshalek P., Dix E., & Sullivan C. (2017). Treatment Outcome Comparison between Telepsychiatry and Face-to-face Buprenorphine Medication-assisted Treatment for Opioid Use Disorder: A 2-Year Retrospective Data Analysis. *Journal of Addiction Medicine*, 11(2), 138-144. https://doi-org.eresources.mssm.edu/10.1097/ADM.0000000000000287.

[8] Ditton P. *Mental Health and Treatment of Inmates and Probationers*. Edited by Dorsey T., Hester T. Washington, DC, Bureau of Justice Statistics, July 1999.

[9] Merideth P. (1999). Forensic applications of telepsychiatry. *Psychiatric Annals*, 29, 429-431. The Royal College of Psychiatrists (RCPsych). (2005). 13th Annual Census of Psychiatric Staffing 2005. http://www.rcpsych.ac.uk/training/census.aspx.

[10] Brodey B. B., Claypoole K. H., Motto J., Arias R. G., Goss R. Satisfaction of forensic psychiatric patients with remote telepsychiatric evaluation. *Psychiatr. Serv.* 2000 Oct; 51(10):1305-7. doi: 10.1176/appi.ps.51.10.1305. PMID: 11013332.

[11] Ferdowsian H., McKenzie K., Zeidan A. Asylum medicine: standard and best practices. *Health and Human Rights Journal*. 2019; 21(1):215-225.

[12] Green A. S., Ruchman S. G., Katz C. L., Singer E. K. Piloting forensic tele-mental health evaluations of asylum seekers. *Psychiatry Res.* 2020 Sep; 291:113256. doi: 10.1016/j.psychres.2020.113256. Epub 2020 Jun 26. PMID: 32619825; PMCID: PMC7319617.

In: Innovations in Psychiatry
Editors: Souparno Mitra et al.
ISBN: 978-1-53619-365-7
© 2021 Nova Science Publishers, Inc.

Chapter 3

APPS FOR ANXIETY

Arun George Prasad, MD*
BronxCare Health System, Department of Psychiatry
Icahn School of Medicine, Bronx, NY, US

ABSTRACT

Anxiety disorders are the most common mental illness in the USA and cause significant morbidity and mortality in the USA. In this chapter we shall discuss apps used for anxiety which are commonly available in the Android/iOS market, and compare their efficacy and individual rating.

INTRODUCTION

Anxiety is the primal physiological response of human beings to help with the fight and flight response ever since evolution. It has become more of a health issue in the past few decades than a natural survival instinct. With society and lifestyle having more of an organized, predictable pattern, with almost no uncertainty regarding where one would get their next meal

---

* Corresponding Author's Email: APrasad1@bronxcare.org.

or find shelter, the human sympathetic response to stress has become more of a mature defense mechanism than a primitive response. Anxiety has become one of the most common and most talked about pathologies of our day. Various theories regarding decreased resilience of the newer generations is a topic that is considered a possible causality [11]. An individualistic approach to life and solo living has empowered people. However, this has also become one of the main reasons for having to deal with life's challenges alone rather than with help from others.

Anxiety disorders are the most common mental illness in the U.S., affecting 40 million adults in the United States age 18 and older, or 18.1% of the population every year. Generalized Anxiety disorder affects 6.8 million adults, or 3.1% of the U.S. population, yet only 43.2% of those affected are receiving treatment [12]. Panic Disorder affects 6 million adults, or 2.7% of the U.S. population. Social Anxiety Disorder affects 15 million adults, or 6.8% of the U.S. population. Specific phobias affect 19 million adults, or 8.7% of the U.S. population. PTSD affects 7.7 million adults, or 3.5% of the U.S. population. The staggering statistics regarding this mental illness goes to show how unaware most people are about the problem, how many cases are going undiagnosed and how much human suffering is being submerged and also the extremely low number of people actually seeking help and being treated. There is no evidence that the prevalence rates of anxiety disorders have changed in the past years, so for decades it has been an undiagnosed health disorder, which has recently come to life more than ever.

ESTABLISHED TREATMENTS FOR ANXIETY

1) Psychotherapeutic Modalities

Cognitive Behavioral Therapy

CBT is typically a short term, skills-focused treatment aimed at altering maladaptive emotional responses by changing thoughts, behaviors or both. It can be used in various subtypes of anxiety disorders including

PTSD, OCD, Panic disorder, Generalized Anxiety disorder, Social anxiety disorder and Specific Phobia. It supposes that changing behaviors leads to changes in emotions and cognitions such as appraisals. It involves assessing automatic thoughts that come up in the context of certain situations in one's life, and the associated Physiological, Psychological and behavioral responses one may present due to them. The core Belief that the patient holds can also be assessed and the theme for most automatic thoughts can be traced from it.

Dialectical Behavioral Therapy

DBT refers to a philosophical practice of examining multiple or often contradictory ideas, combining acceptance and change simultaneously. It has been found to be particularly effective in Parasuicidal patients with Borderline Personality disorder, Women with Borderline personality disorder and a comorbid substance use disorder, Findings indicate that DBT patients had greater reductions in parasuicidal behavior and impulse-control problem behaviors (including bingeing, gambling, and reckless driving, but not substance abuse). The five functions of DBT include- 1) Enhancing capabilities- Improving several important life skills, including those that involve (a) regulating emotions (emotion regulation skills), (b) paying attention to the experience of the present moment and regulating attention (mindfulness skills), (c) effectively navigating interpersonal situations (interpersonal effectiveness), and (d) tolerating distress and surviving crises without making situations worse (distress tolerance skills). 2) Generalizing capabilities, 3) Improving motivation and reducing dysfunctional behaviors. 4) Enhancing and maintaining therapist capabilities and motivation 5) Structuring the environment [13].

Exposure Therapy

It's a type of therapy used mainly in Anxiety disorders in which the therapist gradually exposes an individual to the feared situation in a safe, controlled environment without the intent to cause any harm or danger. A subtype of the therapy is Systemic Desensitization. It is used in treating OCD, phobias, and PTSD. The main aim of the therapy is to reduce the patient's fearful reaction to the stimuli. It can be administered in graded exposure, in which exposure to the feared stimuli is from lower grade to higher grades of exposure levels. Another method is flooding in which the highest intensity of exposure is used right from the start.

Group Therapy

The phrase "group therapy" describes a therapeutic environment with participants beyond a single patient and provider. Multiple people come together and reflect/talk about their symptomatology and their past experience. It has found to be extremely helpful as it shows the patient that they aren't alone and have others who are going through similar experiences, can help each other and find new ways to deal with each other's problems.

2) Pharmacological Therapy

Selective serotonin reuptake inhibitors (SSRIs), serotonin-norepinephrine reuptake inhibitors (SNRIs) and Benzodiazepines are commonly prescribed for Anxiety Disorders.

Table 1. Pharmacotherapy for anxiety disorder

Anxiety Disorder	First-Line Drugs	Second-Line Drugs	Alternatives
Generalized anxiety disorder	Duloxetine Escitalopram Paroxetine Sertraline Venlafaxine XR	Benzodiazepines Buspirone Imipramine Pregabalin	Hydroxyzine Quetiapine
Panic disorder	SSRIs Venlafaxine XR	Alprazolam Citalopram Clomipramine Clonazepam Imipramine	Phenelzine
Social anxiety disorder	Escitalopram Fluvoxamine CR Paroxetine Sertraline Venlafaxine XR	Clonazepam Citalopram	Gabapentin Phenelzine Pregabalin

APPS FOR ANXIETY

As per the data presented above, the majority of the population doesn't seek help for their mental illness. Be it due to a lack of accessibility, inconveniences, lack of time, the taboo of mental illness or financial burdens mental health therapy seems a long way from where it should be. We have heard of the countless celebrities and possibly even people we know who succumb to anxiety and other mental health issues and go as far as committing suicide due to their unmet mental health needs.

Mental health apps can be effective in making therapy more accessible, efficient, and portable, hence making the process of getting help so much easier.

As per the rating scale, mental health apps can be graded on various factors so that individuals can pick apps according to their preferences and find their best match. Apps are often found favorable to those who prefer self- help. They are found to be cost effective and improve the outreach and dissemination of evidence-based mental health care [3].

Some of the main components making mental health apps gradable for efficacy were Psychoeducation, Assessment, Relaxation, Meditation, Mindfulness, Cognitive/Coping, Activity scheduling/Behavioral activation, Self-monitoring, Labelling emotions, Expressing kindness (self), Expressing kindness (to others), Exposure, Modeling, Goal setting, Guided imagery, Stimulus control, Motivational Enhancement, Identifying values, Problem solving, Communication skills, Communication Analysis, Skill Building/Behavioral rehearsal, Homework assignment, Family/Significant other engagement, Behavioral contracting, Assertiveness training [4].

When reviewing online mental health apps, the main components focused on were found to be psychoeducation (in 52% of apps), relaxation (44%), meditation (41%), mindfulness (37%), and assessment (37%) [4].

A compilation of Apps specifically designed for Anxiety with their specific's features are shown below [4].

Table 2. Applications available on the App Store

ApplicationApp Rating (Android/IOS) Downloads Components

- SAM 3.9/4.0500K-1M6
- Simple Habit 4.8/4.7500K-1M6
- Headspace 4.9/4.510M-50M 5
- Mood path 4.7/5.4100K-500K4
- Calm 4.8/4.610M-50M4
- Relax Lite 4.7/3.8500K-1M 3
- Jitters CBT 3.3/NA NA 3
- Rootd 4.1/4.110K-50K 3
- DARE 4.8/4.7100K-500K 1
- Be Okay 4.7/5.0500-10001
- Anxiety Test NA/3.8 50K-100K 1
- End Anxiety Hypnosis NA/4.2 100K-500K 0

As we can see, there are plenty of apps in the market which help with anxiety and depressive disorders. Their popularity varies and efficacy can be assessed by the number of downloads, reviews and feedback submitted by individuals using the apps as well as by controlled trials on these apps with the use of rating scales. Some of the reasons these apps may be becoming popular.

Dearth of Providers

A magnitude of mental health apps exist and are popular because of a serious dearth in mental health resources in the community. According to a 2018 statistic, there are only 9 psychiatrists for every 100,000 people in the US. 60 percent of US counties don't have a single psychiatrist. A majority of these counties are in rural areas. Idaho has less than 1 psychiatrist per 100,000 people, and even in a populous state like Texas, 185 out of 254 counties have no psychiatrists.Talking about urban areas, New York leads the way in Psychiatrist ratio, but still there are only 612 psychiatrists per

100,000 which is still considered underserved [5]. 60 percent of all psychiatrists are over 55 years of age, which makes them the close to retirement. Psychiatry has one of the largest numbers of psychiatrists over the age of 55 years when compared to all other medical specialties [6].

The same goes for psychologists: there are approximately 33.9 Psychologists per 100,000 people in the US, with the lowest being in states like Mississippi (11.9) and South Carolina [13]. [7, 8].

The issue ranges far beyond Psychiatrist/Psychologist availability. The waiting period to see a general psychiatrist could vary from 3 weeks in Los Angeles, to around 3 years to see a child and adolescent psychiatrist in Springfield, Missouri. With such long waiting periods and the need for emergent psychiatric care, the US system has started to rely on Nurse Practitioners and Physician Assistants to deliver Psychiatric care. Another issue we see is cost. Around 45% of psychiatrists didn't accept Medicaid or private health insurance in a 2014 Weill Cornell Medical College study in JAMA Psychiatry that used nationwide data. [9].

New York City private practitioners are known for accepting cash only payments from their rich and elite clients as well as upper-middle class and middle-class clients who are in grave need for Psychiatric care. Their rates vary from 300- 700 dollars for an intake, and 200- 500 dollars for a follow up visit. These rates are simply not affordable for a majority of the population who find relief in cheaper and more accessible mental healthcare online.

Time

This is a factor that has become one of the most important constraints in Modern day living. The corporate lifestyle has made work the #1 priority, and this seldom leaves time for self-care, let alone therapy. Bringing mental health to people's homes via communication devices is a revolutionary idea, and no one can now say "I couldn't find time" to seek mental healthcare ever again.

With so many hurdles and issues the general population faces in acquiring a psychologist/psychiatrist for mental well-being, it is only natural that people go out looking for alternatives and the free market of the West has capitalized on this mass shortage by releasing apps for specific mental health conditions. Easy availability, open and whenever needed access and cheap costs have made them ever so popular on the web.

Many of the apps allow users to start for free, and have up to 10 sessions for free, with a lot of basic content included for free, with an upgrade costs between $4.99 to $19.99 per month, which are more affordable than seeing a Mental Health professional for these acute needs.

Many of these apps have components of cognitive behavioral Therapy, dialectical behavioral therapy, core learning strategies from motivational interviewing, and also just basic techniques like deep breathing and relaxation techniques. Some premium apps have even gone so far as to include live telehealth sessions with trained mental health professionals including Psychologists on demand.

Meditation and mind-fullness apps are booming. The top 10 apps in the market for these are pulling in an estimated $195 Million in 2019, up for 52% compared to 2018. Some newer generation apps are combining journaling, coursework, fitness videos, sleep stories and interviews with celebrities and other inspirational figures to open up on their experiences with anxiety and trauma.

This Multi-Million-dollar industry is starting to make industry experts wonder whether this phenomena on mental health therapy can become a formalized consistent method of delivering mental health services to the under-served and peripheral communities which are in dire need of it.

Some of the most efficient ways to find an app that's suits you would be to do an internet search and find reviews regarding apps and find the one that best suits you or the old school "Word of mouth" regarding the apps.

Some common excerpts from users who have experiences with these apps are included below [10] –

> "I think putting information and expecting it to work for everyone is a bad idea. Personalized is always best because what works for this person may definitely not work for this person as well." This reviewer

states that customizing apps as one uses them is the most efficacious way to utilize an app.

"I think it's nice to have apps that don't require you spending a lot of time on them in one go. You can just dip in and out of them for two or three minutes at a time." A lot of clients with anxiety have attentional problems, catering to the need of shorter attentions spans is essential for app success many believe.

A user in Australia said-

"A lot of times people who are really depressed just don't want to leave the house. They can't be bothered filling up their Opal card [a public transport ticket used in Australia], or catching a bus is too much effort, or they panic. So, there should be a way to access those things within your home."

And then there are the clients who disapproved of the use of technology for therapy-

"If it's too difficult to use an app, I would just uninstall it. There's just so many apps now that if it's too difficult I'll just find another one."
"If you have a mental health app that is also playing music, that is also telling you to exercise, there's like a very small amount of people who will want all those three things in one app."
"I wouldn't recommend someone who's worried to look at this app. It's just too much information bombarded at them" [15, 16].

CONCLUSION

As with Therapists, Mental health apps need to be a perfect fit for the client so that maximum benefit can be derived from them. However, they would never be a one app fits all situation. With the immense competition among these apps in the online free market space, this would only drive the app developers and corporations to keep improving app features with regular updates and always trying to one up each other. With an array of apps available in the market, with free trial periods and features, an informed choice can be made by the millions of subscribers worldwide such that mental health services can be easily accessed sitting in the comforts of their home. Honestly this seems like the golden age of mental health, hopefully with better things to come in the future.

REFERENCES

[1] Gooding, P. A., A. Hurst, J. JohnsonN. Tarrier. *Psychological resilience in young and older adults.* https://doi.org/10.1002/gps.2712.

[2] https://adaa.org/about-adaa/press-room/facts-statistics.

[3] Chapman, Alexander L. PhD. Dialectical Behavior Therapy Current Indications and Unique Elements. *Psychiatry (Edgmont).* 2006 Sep. PMCID: PMC2963469. PMID: 20975829.

[4] Melton, Sarah T. and Cynthia K. Kirkwood Pharmacotherapy A Pathophysiologic Approach, 9th Ed. 53. *Anxiety Disorders I: Generalized Anxiety, Panic, and Social Anxiety Disorders.*

[5] Agras, W. S, Fitzsimmons-Craft, E. E., & Wilfley, D. E (2017). Evolution of cognitive behavioral therapy for eating disorders. Behavior Research and Therapy. American Psychiatric Association. (n.d). *App. evaluation model.* Retrieved from www.psychiatry.org/psychiatrists/practice/mental-health-apps/app-evalua tionmodel.

[6] Akash R. Wasil, Katherine E. Venturo-Conerly, Rebecca M. Shingleton, John R. Weisz. *A review of popular smart phone apps for depression and anxiety: Assessing the inclusion of evidence-based content.*

[7] *"The Silent Shortage: How Immigration Can Address the Large and Growing Psychiatrist Shortage in the United States"* www.newameri

caneconomy.org/wp-content/uploads/2017/10/NAE_Psychiatrist Shortage_V6-1.pdf.

[8] National Council for Behavioral Health. *Press Release: Medical Directors' Report Recommends Training More Psychiatrists and Expanding Telepsychiatry.* Washington, DC, March 28, 2017. Available at: https://www.thenationalcouncil.org/wp-content/uploads/2016/11/Access-paper-release-final-3.28.17-final.pdf.

[9] American Psychological Association (2014). 2012 *APA state licensing board list.* [Unpublished special analysis]. Washington, DC: Author.

[10] U. S. Census Bureau. (2012). *Annual estimates of the Resident Population for the United States, Regions, States, and Puerto Rico*: April 1, 2010, to July 1, 2012. Retrieved from http://www.census.gov/popest/data/historical/2010s/vintage_2012/state.html.

[11] American Psychological Association. *About Prescribing Psychologists.* Available at: www.apaservices.org/practice/advocacy/authority/prescribing-psychologists. Accessed October 8, 2019.

[12] Sandra Garrido, Daniel Cheers, Katherine Boydell, Quang Vinh Nguyen, Emery Schubert, Laura Dunne, Tanya Meade. *JMIR Ment Health.* 2019 Oct; 6(10): e14385. doi: 10.2196/14385. PMID: 31579023.

[13] Anxiety: There is an app for that. *A systematic review of anxiety apps* Madalina Sucala PhD, Pim Cuijpers PhD, Frederick Muench PhD, Roxana Cardoş PhD, Radu Soflau PhD, Anca Dobrean PhD, Patriciu Achimas-Cadariu PhD, Daniel David PhD. https://doi-org.eresources.mssm.edu/10.1002/da.22654.

[14] *Young People's Response to Six Smartphone Apps for Anxiety and Depression: Focus Group Study JMIR Ment Health.* 2019 Oct; 6(10): e14385. Published online 2019 Oct 2. doi: 10.2196/14385, PMCID: PMC6915797. PMID: 31579023.

[15] National Institute of Mental Health and *World Health Organization: Mental Health.* https://adaa.org/about-adaa/press-room/facts-statistic.

[16] ADAA Reviewed Mental Health Apps, *Anxiety and Depression Association of America.*

In: Innovations in Psychiatry
Editors: Souparno Mitra et al.
ISBN: 978-1-53619-365-7
© 2021 Nova Science Publishers, Inc.

Chapter 4

JOURNALING APPS

Maria Alejandra Gallo-Ruiz, MD*

BronxCare Health System, Department of Psychiatry,
Icahn School of Medicine, Bronx, NY, US

ABSTRACT

Journals have been used for documents, thoughts and feelings for aeons. With the advent of smartphones, journaling applications have been developed and people have been able to document their thoughts and feelings in real-time. In our chapter, we will discuss the different options of applications that are available for use in journaling and the different kinds of journaling that do exist.

INTRODUCTION

With the increased involvement of the internet and everything that it brings with itself into people's lives, it is not a surprise that it has found its way into the field of mental health. It can be said that it has made some

---

* Corresponding Author's Email: MRuiz@bronxcare.org.

tools more easily available, and people may be more ready to use them on this platform. In this chapter we are going to review a well-known activity for everyone that lately has been actively used for mental health treatment modalities. We are talking about the very simple activity of writing down one's' feelings, emotions and daily thoughts, more commonly known as "journaling."

People may consider journaling to be similar to the childhood activity of maintaining a diary. And even if we didn't try it, we heard of it. The positive outcomes of journaling in people's daily living have been studied, and journaling has been associated with decreased mental distress and increase in subjective feeling of well-being with decreased anxiety and depressive symptoms.

TYPES OF JOURNALS

Few people may be aware of this, but journaling has different types which are as follows:

- Reflective Journaling

Reflective journaling refers to journaling which requires the participant to write and reflect upon experiences you deem profound or that have had an impact on your life. So it is done to express the event, think about the significance it had and what you may have learned from it. In this form of journaling it is important to write as soon as possible so you won't forget details.

Some of the common reasons to use it include:

o To make sense of things that happened, writing as in much detail as possible may give you a different perspective that you didn't consider before.

Journaling Apps

- o   To speculate as to why something is the way it is.
- o   To align future actions with your reflected values.
- o   To get thoughts out of your head.

- Gratitude Journaling

It is a record of things you appreciate or are thankful for. It can be material things, good things that happened to you or to reflect on how to express gratitude to others. Or can help you to reflect in maybe some no so good situations but the good things they may have emerge from it in your life.

Some of the common reasons to use it include:

- o   It helps to keep your priorities organized, keeping a record of what we are grateful for, gives you the opportunity to know what matters to you and with this you can gain insight on what to spend more time and energy on.
- o   It helps you to correct your perspective when it is skewed
- o   It can help you in rough patches when life seems difficult
- o   It helps you to have a more positive outlook in life.
- o   and talking about challenges, obstacles in life may have given us the opportunity to develop a part of our identity that later we can be proud of.

- Goal Planning Journals

These involve writing about what you would like to accomplish in different areas of your life in terms of career, spirituality, family, activism and hobbies. Depending on the goal, you may have a checklist with a small writing area or prompts giving you tasks to complete and thoughts regarding those tasks.

Most common reasons to use it include:

- o It helps you to conceptualize your goals, organize your schedule, and overcome procrastination in a structured way.
- o It can help you create healthy habits.
- o It can help you achieve your goals by organizing them in a timeline and small steps.

- Specialized Journals (Dream Journal, Art Journal, Prayer Journal, etc.)

Lastly, you can use journaling to focus on a specific topic. There are various journals available that focus on a specific topic. You may want to start a dream journal so that you can start to remember your dreams better. You may want to start an art journal if drawing is something that you enjoy or if it helps you work through thoughts and emotions. Some people keep prayer journals or bible journals, where you can write and reflect about specific passages.

After you decide what kind of journal you are most interested in, you can choose that journal and start writing in it. The most important thing is to understand that your journal is in many ways a dialogue that you are having with yourself.

You are forcing your brain to think critically and to produce written words accordingly; there is no need to pay careful attention to spelling or grammar. A thing that may be important or useful is to keep your journal nearby. Using mobile phone apps are a huge help in this regard. Better results can be seen if you make regular entries, this ensures you are actively thinking and enables critical thinking. Lastly, try to review your journal regularly, it can help reflect on how far you have come and can be of most help when you are having a hard day so you can see the progress you made which can sometimes be difficult to see when changes are subtle.

Journaling in the Era of the Internet

Now we are going to review journaling in the internet era, which essentially means the use of journaling apps. A paper and pen are perfectly fine for journaling, but apps can offer more. They sometimes may be more easily available, because we all know that the majority of the population carries a phone with them at all times. Apps are more interactive, and you can include photos from your phone or posts from your social media feeds to make the journaling experience more rewarding. You can set up reminders if that is something that can make things easier for you and it also gives you the opportunity to look for past entries in an easier way.

Characteristic of Ideal Journaling Apps

The characteristics that you should look for in a journaling app are:

- Easy entry: the least you struggle doing it, higher the chances you will really do it.
- Pleasant interface: clean organized presentation, that provides what is just necessary for you to write.
- Reminders: Until you make it a habit, reminders will keep you on track.
- Syncing: this can be a plus so you can use it in different devices, if this is something you are interested in.

APPLICATIONS AVAILABLE FOR USE ON COMPUTERS AND SMARTPHONES

The following list is a collection of applications available on the Android, iOS and Windows platforms for journaling:

1. Day One: Best Rated App for Apple

It is one of the highest rated apps on the Apple Store and it's not hard to see why. The app offers a wide array of features. You can create journal entries in just one click on the Mac from the menu bar, use templates to make journaling easier, and automatically add metadata, such as location, weather, motion activity, currently playing music, and step count. You can also tag entries with hashtags, insert photos and videos, password-protect your journal, and format entries in Markdown. And all of this is within an elegant, unobtrusive design. It also gives you the option to customize multiple reminders.

2. Diarium. Best journal App for Windows Users

Diarium stands out for its support for multiple media types in journal entries. If you'd rather speak than type, you can dictate your thoughts with accurate speech recognition. You can attach an audio file, inked drawing, or any other type of file to your entries, as well as multiple photos. You can even rate your journal entries (perhaps most useful as a way to track how happy you are each day).

Diarium syncs to other Windows devices or Android with OneDrive. You can also export your entries to DOCX, HTML, RTF, or TXT formats - with separate files for media attachments - so you can rest assured that your data will always be accessible. We found the syncing between Windows and Android instant and reliable.

3. Journey. Best Journal App for Cross-Platform Journaling

Journey is the one journaling app that was found to work across pretty much any platform. And it does it well, with features that rival those of the other top journaling app picks. Standouts include support for multiple images, as well as audio or video exporting to multiple formats, auto location and weather, and password protection.

4. Penzu. Best Journal App for Secure Journaling

Penzu comes with a very simple and convenient design. Penzu keeps your entries together in one journal online, as opposed to several different files. Custom email reminders help you remember to record your journal entry. Also, Penzu can send you reminders of what you've written in the past so that you can reminisce about the good old days.

More importantly, Penzu will keep your entries 100 percent private. You can lock your journal with a special password, secure your content with 128-bit encryption, and choose to auto-lock your journal at all times. If you're on the Pro plan, Penzu can safeguard your entries with military-strength 256-bit encryption.

5. Momento. Best Journal App for Social Media Power Users

Momento brings all of your shared posts and interactions from sites into one place, helping you keep a digital archive of your online interactions. Momento supports 11 feeds, including your Uber trip history, Spotify saved tracks, and YouTube videos. You can also create new journal entries like you would with a typical journaling app.

Momento excels at resurfacing where you've been and what you've done in the past. You can group separate entries (or "moments") into "events" - so all of the Instagram photos you were tagged in for a family reunion could live together. The app will show you what happened on a specific date in previous years, so you can see how time has flown. It also presets reminders: for example, "what did you dream?" at 7:30 am and "how was your day?" at 8 pm - make it easier to journal when you're not sure what to write.

6. Grid Diary. Best Journal App for Templated Journaling

Every day, the app presents you with eight question prompts, such as "What sports did I do today to improve my health?," "What have I done with my family today," and "What can I do today to make my future better," laid out on a one-page grid. This gives you a detailed and bird's eye view of what's happening in your life, one day at a time.

There are numerous grid templates you can choose from or you can customize the grid and questions yourself to focus on the areas of life you want to track. Instead of wondering what you should write about each day, you can use Grid Diary to write down simple responses that help you reflect on your days.

7. Five-Minute Journal. Best Journal App for Beginners

Five Minute Journal makes journaling easy and approachable with timed prompts throughout the day. In the morning, the app asks you three questions designed to instill gratitude and set a purpose for your day. In the evening, two questions ask you to reflect on the positive things that happened and how you could improve for tomorrow.

Based on positive psychology research, Five Minute Journal helps support a gratitude habit and self-reflection. You can add a photo for each entry and export to PDF, but if you're looking for a freeform journaling app to write as much as you want, this isn't the app for you.

8. Daylio. Best Journal App for Non-Writers

If you prefer to communicate in visuals, Daylio is the app for you.

A journal entry in Daylio captures your mood and activities for each day. Best of all, there is absolutely no typing, but you are welcome to do it too, if that is what you want. Pick your mood by selecting one of five smiley face icons. You can choose particular icons for what you were up to during that day. Both the mood options and activities can be customized. While it takes just a few seconds to complete each entry, the details add up to form a well-rounded picture of what your day was like.

Daylio also includes standard journaling features, like reminders, exporting entries, and setting goals. As a bonus, it offers a detailed dashboard that aggregates a monthly mood chart, your mood and activity counts, and average daily mood. It can also surface patterns in the "Often together" section, showing you how you usually feel when you do certain activities (for example, when your mood is "good," you usually exercise and spend time in nature).

In this chapter, we wanted to give you the different options of types of journaling and the different apps that can help you to do it, now you have all the tools to start, Good Luck!.

CASE STUDY

Julie is a 27-year-old art master's student. Three months ago she started feeling low and was finding it difficult to get motivated to meet deadlines. At the beginning, she just took it as a momentary rough patch. Over the next few weeks, she began struggling more and more with motivation and everything seemed like a huge effort. She began having self-deprecating thoughts like "I am stuck in a rut," "Everyone else is doing better than me," "I'm going no-where." Things she previously really enjoyed doing like swimming and seeing her friends were no longer enjoyable.

Since everything was such an effort for Julie, and when she did make the effort, she didn't enjoy it, she began doing less and less. Her friends called regularly and invited her out, but she started to refuse these invitations because she no longer enjoyed being out socially and she felt like a burden on her friends. By the end of February, Julie was no longer going out other than for work, she was struggling to get out of bed in the morning and when she was at work, she found everything took a huge effort and she thought everything she produced was "useless." She began to feel hopeless about the future, her mood became lower and she decided to take two weeks off to "try and sort herself out."

She went to her primary care physician, during the visit, she was very shy and quiet and was not able to explain in detail to her doctor what was going on since she had an overwhelming feeling of guilt and embarrassment from thinking that she was struggling without any "real problems going on." Julie's doctor was able to see through her pain, he recommended her to write a journal for 2 week about her concerns and feelings to be reviewed in a further visit. Julie went back home feeling guilty of being unable to talk to her doctor but followed her doctor recommendations. At the beginning she just spend a few minutes a day writing a few words, but then she started noticing that writing facilitated for her to connect to her feelings and how thinking about her feelings felt a bit like a release and she kept coming back to it as a way to process what was happening in her life, she came back to her doctor and she didn't even had to show the journal to her doctor, she just was able to articulate in words what was happening in her life for so long, her doctor listen to her and recommended an antidepressant but firmly recommended to keep writing in her journal. Julie kept her doctor's recommendations and started working again, initially was very hard for her but with time everything went back to place, she was able to start spending time with family and friends, and even kept journaling after stopping medications.

Conclusion

Journaling has always been a popular treatment modality. With the advent of the internet, e-journaling applications may be what we need to enable greater efficacy, compliance and interpretation of data.

References

[1] Apple Store.
[2] Google Play Store.

In: Innovations in Psychiatry
Editors: Souparno Mitra et al.
ISBN: 978-1-53619-365-7
© 2021 Nova Science Publishers, Inc.

Chapter 5

C-CBT

Aditya Sareen[*]*, MD and Bibiana Susaimanickam, MD*

BronxCare Health System, Department of Psychiatry Icahn School of Medicine, Bronx, NY, US

Abstract

Cognitive behavioral therapy (CBT) is an evidence-based treatment modality used to treat depression, anxiety, stress, eating disorders, post-traumatic stress disorder (PTSD) and related mental challenges. CBT actively engages the patient in addressing these issues by learning new ways of thinking, feeling and behaving that promote improved self-care and mental wellness.

With the advent of the internet and mobile devices, increasingly, mental health organizations are offering an online version of this approach called "computerized CBT" or c- CBT. As the demand for mental health services increases, providers are seeking new ways to assist larger population in the most efficient manner. The c-CBT approach directly addresses this need. In this chapter we discuss about advantages and limitations of c-CBT and its utilization specifically in treatment of depression, anxiety, insomnia and eating disorders.

---

[*] Corresponding Author's Email: ASareen@bronxcare.org.

INTRODUCTION

Cognitive Behavioral Therapy (CBT) is a form of psychological treatment that has demonstrated to be effective for a range of problems including depression, anxiety, eating disorders, drug problems and severe mental illness. In the past the only way to deliver CBT was through a face to face individual contact to the clinician. However the past couple of decades have seen a rise of computers and mobile phones, which in turn has led to easy accessibility for individuals to have a face to face interaction with others over video conferencing.

The availability and use of computers, the Internet, and mobile phones have expanded tremendously. In 2019, nearly 90% of U.S. adults accessed the Internet and 81% of U.S. adults had a smartphone, up from 35% in 2011(pewresearch.org). As access has grown so has the functionality of technology and at the same time, technological advances have become less expensive, more compact, and more powerful [25].

A computer or a mobile phone with such features can be used to exchange information and a means of communication between the health care professionals and patients for administrative or therapeutic purposes. Such advances have paved the way for delivery of CBT through these mediums called computerized- Cognitive Behavioral Therapy (c-CBT).

c-CBT can be delivered by a number of methods using an interactive interface (via a mobile phone or a computer) that uses patient input to make some psychotherapy decisions. It can be used as the primary treatment intervention with minimal therapist involvement or as an adjunct to a therapist delivered program. At present c-CBT has been primarily used for individuals with anxiety disorders such as panic disorder, phobias, social anxiety, post-traumatic stress disorder and obsessive-compulsive disorder and mild to moderate depression. There is also some evidence of the use of c-CBT in eating disorders, sexual disorders, psychosis, substance abuse treatment, alcohol, smoking cessation among others. c-CBT has also been used for several health conditions such as pain, tinnitus, insomnia, breast cancer etc. [1].

c-CBT has several advantages such as its capacity to deliver structured input consistently with precision, low cost, easy accessibility and flexibility in a non-stigmatized environment [2].

This enables c-CBT to be available for more people in an efficient manner and can be delivered in any suitable environment even at home. c-CBT offers more control to the client promoting agency, mastery, control and learned resourcefulness [3]. Whereas, non-electronic CBT, have several problems which include increased cost, long waiting times for therapy, inadequate access to the services and an unequal geographic distribution of accredited CBT therapist [4]. A recent meta-analysis in 2020 by Luo et al, compared the effects of c-CBT compared to face-to-face CBT through a systematic review of the literature. They found 17 studies which demonstrated that c-CBT was more effective than face-to-face CBT at reducing depression symptom severity and there were no significant differences between the two interventions on participant satisfaction.

There are also potential drawbacks of c-CBT such as lack of face-to-face contact, privacy and safety issues. A systematic review on the acceptability of c-CBT in depression was conducted in 2008. The authors found that limited information was provided on patient take-up rates and recruitment methods. Drop-out rates were comparable to other forms of treatment. Take-up rates, where much lower. Six of the 16 studies included specific questions on patient acceptability or satisfaction although information was only provided for those who had completed treatment [5]. A recent trial (REEACT trial) in 2015 evaluated the clinical effectiveness and cost effectiveness of c-CBT as an adjunct to usual general practitioner care against general practitioner care alone using a free to use c-CBT program (MoodGYM) and a pay to use c-CBT program (Beating the blues) for the treatment of depression in primary care. They found that that neither of the c-CBT program (Beating the Blues nor MoodGYM) appeared cost-effective compared with usual GP care alone [6].

A newer technology has also emerged called Cognitive Bias Modification (CBM) which is also deployed through a computer. In this technique individuals are not required to engage in reflective thinking about their own thought patterns (as in c-CBT), CBM instead erodes threat-related cognitive biases by repeated computer-based practice in disengaging from threat-related stimuli using a visual probe task (cognitive bias modification for attention; CBM-A), or interpreting emotional ambiguity in a positive direction (cognitive bias modification for interpretation; CBM-I). Bowler et al, compared the c-CBT to CBM-I and found that both CBM-I and c-CBT groups reported significantly reduced levels of social anxiety, trait anxiety, and depression and improved attentional control, relative to the control group, with no clear superiority of either active intervention. Although both active conditions reduced negative bias on the Scrambled Sentences Test completed under mental load, CBM-I was significantly more effective at doing so [7].

In conclusion, there is a growing evidence and support of the use of c-CBT in several mental health problems. Further research is required in evaluation of the effectiveness and acceptability of c-CBT. A consideration should be made regarding the privacy and safety of information shared through such platforms.

C-CBT USE IN DEPRESSION

A number of studies have shown efficacy of c-CBT for the treatment of Depression. c-CBT combined with modest amounts of clinician support, offers potential for delivery of evidence-based treatment at greater efficiency and lower cost than standard CBT [8].

A Meta review of effectiveness of C-CBT in treatment of depression found limited evidence of effectiveness of three C-CBT applications (MoodGYM, Beating the Blues and Colour Your Life), but not enough of such evidence to prefer one package for depression over another. However this meta analysis does not take onto consideration the two large pragmatic trials The Randomized Evaluation of the Effectiveness and Acceptability of Computerized Therapy (REEACT) Trial and computerized CBT for Common Mental Disorders: RCT of a Workplace Intervention.

The Randomized Evaluation of the Effectiveness and Acceptability of computerized Therapy (REEACT) Trial was a pragmatic, multi-center, three arm, parallel randomized controlled trial with simple randomization to receive a commercially produced c-CBT program ("Beating the Blues") or a free to use c-CBT program (MoodGYM) in patients with depression, in addition to usual general physician (GP) care. 691 participants were enrolled in this study. They found Computerized cognitive behavior therapy had modest or no benefit over usual GP care and suggests that the routine promotion and commissioning of c-CBT be reconsidered in light of our findings. Commercially developed computerized cognitive behavior therapy products confer little or no benefit over free to use products. This appears to be an important finding for those who commission services and purchase commercial products on behalf of publicly funded health services. The routine use and purchase of computerized therapy is likely to be an ineffective form of low intensity treatment for depression and an inefficient use of finite healthcare resources [10].

A second Randomized Evaluation of the Effectiveness and Acceptability of computerized Therapy (REEACT-2) was conducted to compare the clinical effectiveness and cost-effectiveness of telephone-facilitated free-to-use c-CBT (e.g., MoodGYM) with minimally supported c-CBT. This was also a multisite, pragmatic, open, two-arm, parallel-group randomized controlled trial. 182 participants were randomized to minimally supported c-CBT and 187 participants to telephone-facilitated c-CBT. They concluded that there were short-term benefits from the addition of telephone facilitation to c-CBT. The effect was small to moderate and comparable with that of other primary care psychological interventions. Therefore, telephone facilitation should be considered when offering c-CBT for depression [11].

Computerized CBT for Common Mental Disorders: RCT of a Workplace Intervention was a phase III two-arm, parallel randomized controlled trial whose was to investigate the effectiveness of a computerized CBT intervention (MoodGYM) in a workplace context. The main outcome was total score on the Work and Social Adjustment Scale (WSAS). Depression, anxiety, psychological functioning, costs and acceptability of the online process were also measured. They found no evidence that MoodGYM was superior to informational websites in terms of psychological outcomes or service use, although improvement to subthreshold levels of depression was seen in nearly half the patients in both groups [12].

C-CBT USE IN ANXIETY DISORDERS

CBT has been used widely and effectively for the treatment of Anxiety disorders and now c-CBT has also been intervention that has been used for these disorders [1].

Studies by Proudfoot et al. 2004 [18] show that with a larger sample size for the treatment of patients with anxiety and/ or depression with c-CBT programs had led to significant improvement in most variables measured in the study including – decrease in depression and anxiety, work and social adjustment improved, negative attributions decreased, positive attributions increased and satisfaction with treatment was enhanced. These effects were substantial as well as statistically significant. They were noted to be effective even for patient with moderate to severe symptoms, similar to those observed by Miranda & Munoz, 1994.

It was also noted that for patients with anxiety, c-CBT also led to greater satisfaction with treatment. They concluded that c-CBT is clinically effective in the treatment of anxiety, depression and mixed anxiety/depression in general practice. The specific program studied, *Beating the Blues*, is widely applicable in general practice, and its efficacy over a 6-month follow-up period was unaffected by age, gender, concomitant drug treatment or duration of pre-existing illness.

With limitation outlined as that the outcomes were measured by self-report. The patients were not masked to treatment (necessarily so, given its nature). Some data were missing (a frequent hazard in naturalistic research).

Other studies have noted limitations due to lack of face-to-face contact and potential issues relating to safety. Additionally, supported c-CBT interventions have higher rates of adherence and better outcomes than unsupported programs, and services can provide support for c-CBT to improve the benefits of these programs. This support might include information and taster sessions of c-CBT programs to promote uptake along with regular support offered face-to-face, by phone or email and log-on reminders to promote program engagement, adherence and completion [22].

Newby et al. 2016, [19] in their study discussed about computerized transdiagnostic cognitive behavioral therapy programs (TD-c-CBT) have been developed in the past decade.

This meta-analysis focused on studies evaluating TD-c-CBT interventions to examine their effects on anxiety, depression and quality of life (QOL). Results from 17 RCTs showed computerized TD-c-CBT outperformed control conditions on all outcome measures at post-treatment, with large effect sizes for depression and medium effect sizes for anxiety and QOL RCT quality was generally good, although heterogeneity was moderate to high. Treatment length, symptom target (mixed versus anxiety only), treatment design (standardized versus tailored), and therapist experience (students versus qualified therapists) did not influence the results. Preliminary evidence from 4 comparisons with disorder-specific treatments suggests transdiagnostic treatments are as effective for reducing anxiety, and there may be small but superior outcomes for TD-c-CBT programs for reducing depression and improving QOL compared to disorder-specific c-CBT. These findings show that TD-c-CBT programs are efficacious, and have comparable effects to disorder-specific c-CBT programs.

In a recent meta-analysis done on the effectiveness of c-CBT [23] found it to be beneficial for reducing post-treatment anxiety and depressive symptoms in adolescents and young adults compared with passive controls. Compared with active treatment controls, c-CBT yielded similar effects regarding anxiety symptoms. In this study though regarding depressive symptoms, the results remain unclear. There was recommendations for more high-quality research involving active controls and long-term follow-up assessments in this population.

Overall, there is growing interest and an expanding evidence base for c-CBT in the management of common mental health problems

C-CBT USE IN INSOMNIA

Insomnia is estimated to affect 9%-15% of the world's population [15]. Notably, the relationship between insomnia and depression is bi-directional; individuals with insomnia are at significantly higher risk of developing depression, and persons with depression are at higher risk of developing insomnia [13]. While insomnia is of major public health importance, its treatment predominantly occurs in primary care and outpatient mental health settings, with cognitive behavioral therapy for insomnia (CBTI) often offered as a first-line therapy in adults. The American Academy of Sleep Medicine recommends CBTI for chronic primary insomnia disorder with and without comorbid conditions [14].

However as beneficial as cognitive behavioral therapy is for the treatment of insomnia, in-person CBTI is not easily accessible to all individuals with insomnia. There is a lack of well-trained therapists specializing in CBTI to fill the need [15].

Studies like Seyffert et al. 2016 have done metanalysis to see online cognitive behavioral therapy for insomnia could improve sleep efficiency and reduce the severity of insomnia in adults. They showed that Sleep efficiency was 72% at baseline and improved by 7.2% (95% CI: 5.1%, 9.3%; p<0.001) with internet-delivered cognitive behavioral therapy versus control. Internet-delivered cognitive behavioral therapy resulted in a decrease in the insomnia severity index by 4.3 points (95% CI: -7.1, -1.5; p = 0.017) compared to control. Improvements in sleep efficiency, the insomnia severity index and depression scores with internet-delivered cognitive behavioral therapy were maintained from 4 to 48 weeks after post-treatment assessment [16].

Since persons with various mental disorders often experience insomnia, access to internet-delivered CBTI may provide flexibility and convenience (e.g., in those that suffer social anxiety or agoraphobia).

Additionally, internet-delivered CBTI holds the potential to improve access to insomnia treatment for individuals with limited transportation options or those that live in rural areas and cannot physically access a trained therapist.

Internet-based mental health platforms are already approved by the National Health Service in the United Kingdom as part of a stepped care approach, with internet-delivered CBTI recommended as one of the options for individuals with sub-threshold symptoms and those with certain mental health disorders [17].

Some limitations found this metanalysis was no control group to study the adverse effect of sleep restriction therapy, a component of CBTI. For future studies using CBTI, it is important that any adverse effects are measured (similar to any other randomized controlled trial) and that proper controls with insomnia are utilized so that the background rate of effects can be compared.

Additional trials that more fully delineate the most effective features of internet engagement may be informative, as well as whether supplemental aids or assistance would provide benefits.

C-CBT USE IN EATING DISORDERS

Cognitive behavioral therapy (CBT) is an evidence-based treatment for bulimia nervosa and binge-eating disorder (BED) and is regarded as the first-line treatment for both eating disorders (ED). The general consensus is that CBT is more effective than other psychotherapies in the treatment of Bulimia Nervosa (BN) and should, therefore, be the preferred psychotherapeutic treatment [27]. Moreover, the research literature has some notable strengths including the development of detailed treatment manuals, standardization of outcome measures particularly the use of the

Eating Disorder Examination (EDE), comparisons of CBT with other active treatments rather than waitlist controls, and the use of multisite studies. With the rise of technology, CBT for eating disorders has also seen advances.

A systemic literature review [26] found that internet-based treatments were superior to waiting lists in reducing ED psychopathology, frequency of binge eating and purging, and in improving (ED-related) quality of life. Internet-based treatment was more effective for individuals with less comorbid psychopathology, binge eating as opposed to restrictive problems, and individuals with binge eating disorder as opposed to bulimia nervosa. Higher levels of compliance were related to more improvements in ED symptoms. Inclusion of face-to-face assessments and therapist support seemed to enhance study compliance.

It is also important to note due to medical co-morbidities associated with BN, medical screening prior to entry into treatment is needed, and for Anorexia Nervosa (AN) medical screening and ongoing medical monitoring is essential. Medical history, physical examination to the extent needed, and necessary blood tests should be obtained for controlled treatment studies including Internet therapy. Such medical clearance could be assessed either at the study site or by the participant's family physician who would then provide written clearance for participation. Lack of medical follow up may act as a limitation in the delivery of care. Two of the Internet-based studies described the use of a medical examination together with appropriate blood tests prior to study entry [28, 29].

Detection of comorbid pathologies is also important given the high prevalence of such disorders in bulimic syndromes. This would be the usual standard of care for a clinical consultation. Acceptable forms of face-to-face assessment beyond a direct interview might be via Skype or teleconference. In addition, some method of monitoring comorbid psychopathology throughout treatment should be instigated so that changes throughout therapy can be followed. Consideration should be given to withdrawing participants who show lack of progress or worsening of primary or comorbid psychopathology and providing specialized care. Lack of medical follow up may act as a limitation in the delivery of care.

Analyses for the individual subgroups BN, BED, and ED NOS showed that eating disorder psychopathology improved significantly over time among Web-based CBT participants in all three subgroups; however, the between-group effect was significant only for participants with BED [24].

CONCLUSION

In this era of surviving a pandemic and providing optimized care for patients in a safe manner, telehealth services is going to play a vital role. Therefore, using computers and/or internet to treat patients with evidence-based modalities like CBT is all the more vital.

It has numerous purported benefits including: lack of geographic boundaries, allowing for widespread dissemination and the ability to reach individuals who may otherwise have limited access to effective treatment (e.g., those in rural communities) or who may not seek help due to shame or fear of stigma; easy access from anywhere at any time; cost and time efficient; enhancing health literacy and high user acceptability [30]. In the meantime being mindful of safety, healthy patient boundaries and insurance coverage of services; ensuring that there is less drop offs from the programs.

Telehealth is ultimately a system of systems in scale and complexity. Overall, end-user adoption is challenged by the need for the integration of new technologies in clinical practice workflow and daily activities. Adoption requires cultural and behavioral changes for use and reliance on telehealth technologies. From the patient's perspective, the usability and ease-of-access to technologies are obstructed by the lack of technology integration, interoperability, and standardization. The key will be to putting the "person "in "personalized medicine" [31].

REFERENCES

[1] Marks, I. M., & Gega, L. (2009). Review by Jeroen Ruwaard and Alfred Lange (Cognitive Behaviour Therapy, 2009, 38(2), p. 132) of Hands-on-Help: Computer-Aided Psychotherapy (Maudsley Monograph 49) by I. M. Marks, K. Cavanagh, and L. Gega. New York: Psychology Press 2007. Letter to the editors. *Cognitive behaviour therapy*, 38(3), 192. https://doi.org/10.1080/16506070903162889.

[2] Foroushani, P. S., Schneider, J., & Assareh, N. (2011). Meta-review of the effectiveness of computerised CBT in treating depression. *BMC psychiatry*, 11, 131. https://doi.org/10.1186/1471-244X-11-131.

[3] Kaltenthaler, E. and Cavanagh, K. (2010), Computerised cognitive behavioural therapy and its uses. *Prog. Neurol. Psychiatry,* 14: 22-29. doi: 10.1002/pnp.163.

[4] Cavanagh K. (2014). Geographic inequity in the availability of cognitive behavioural therapy in England and Wales: a 10-year update. *Behavioural and cognitive psychotherapy*, 42(4), 497–501. https://doi.org/10.1017/S1352465813000568.

[5] Kaltenthaler, E., Sutcliffe, P., Parry, G., Beverley, C., Rees, A., & Ferriter, M. (2008). The acceptability to patients of computerized cognitive behaviour therapy for depression: a systematic review. *Psychological medicine*, 38(11), 1521–1530. https://doi-org.eresources.mssm.edu/10.1017/S0033291707002607.

[6] Littlewood, E., Duarte, A., Hewitt, C., Knowles, S., Palmer, S., Walker, S., Andersen, P., Araya, R., Barkham, M., Bower, P., Brabyn, S., Brierley, G., Cooper, C., Gask, L., Kessler, D., Lester, H., Lovell, K., Muhammad, U., Parry, G., Richards, D. A., … REEACT Team (2015). A randomised controlled trial of computerised cognitive behaviour therapy for the treatment of depression in primary care: The Randomised Evaluation of the Effectiveness and Acceptability of Computerised Therapy

(REEACT) trial. *Health technology assessment (Winchester, England)*, 19(101), viii–171. https://doi.org/10.3310/hta191010.

[7] Bowler, J. O., Mackintosh, B., Dunn, B. D., Mathews, A., Dalgleish, T., & Hoppitt, L. (2012). A comparison of cognitive bias modification for interpretation and computerized cognitive behavior therapy: effects on anxiety, depression, attentional control, and interpretive bias. *Journal of consulting and clinical psychology*, *80*(6), 1021–1033. https://doi-org.eresources.mssm.edu/10.1037/a0029932.

[8] Wright J. H., Owen J. J., Richards D., Eells T. D., Richardson T., Brown G. K., Barrett M., Rasku M. A., Polser G., Thase M. E. Computer-Assisted Cognitive-Behavior Therapy for Depression: A Systematic Review and Meta-Analysis. *J Clin Psychiatry.* 2019 Mar 19;80(2):18r12188. doi: 10.4088/JCP.18r12188. PMID: 30900849.

[9] Foroushani, P. S., Schneider, J., & Assareh, N. (2011). Meta-review of the effectiveness of computerised CBT in treating depression. *BMC psychiatry*, 11, 131. https://doi.org/10.1186/1471-244X-11-131.

[10] Littlewood, E., Duarte, A., Hewitt, C., Knowles, S., Palmer, S., Walker, S., Andersen, P., Araya, R., Barkham, M., Bower, P., Brabyn, S., Brierley, G., Cooper, C., Gask, L., Kessler, D., Lester, H., Lovell, K., Muhammad, U., Parry, G., Richards, D. A., ... REEACT Team (2015). A randomised controlled trial of computerised cognitive behaviour therapy for the treatment of depression in primary care: the Randomised Evaluation of the Effectiveness and Acceptability of Computerised Therapy (REEACT) trial. *Health technology assessment (Winchester, England)*, 19(101), viii–171. https://doi.org/10.3310/hta191010.

[11] Brabyn, S., Araya, R., Barkham, M., Bower, P., Cooper, C., Duarte, A., Kessler, D., Knowles, S., Lovell, K., Littlewood, E., Mattock, R., Palmer, S., Pervin, J., Richards, D., Tallon, D., White, D., Walker, S., Worthy, G., & Gilbody, S. (2016). The second Randomised Evaluation of the Effectiveness, cost-effectiveness and Acceptability of Computerised Therapy (REEACT-2) trial: does the provision of

telephone support enhance the effectiveness of computer-delivered cognitive behaviour therapy? A randomised controlled trial. *Health technology assessment (Winchester, England)*, 20(89), 1–64. https://doi.org/10.3310/hta20890.

[12] Phillips, R., Schneider, J., Molosankwe, I., Leese, M., Foroushani, P. S., Grime, P., McCrone, P., Morriss, R., & Thornicroft, G. (2014). Randomized controlled trial of computerized cognitive behavioural therapy for depressive symptoms: effectiveness and costs of a workplace intervention. *Psychological medicine,* 44(4), 741–752. https://doi.org/10.1017/S0033291713001323.

[13] Sivertsen B., Salo P., Mykletun A., Hysing M., Pallesen S., Krokstad S., et al. The bidirectional association between depression and insomnia: the HUNT study. *Psychosom Med.* 2012; 74(7):758–765. 10.1097/PSY.0b013e3182648619.

[14] Schutte-Rodin S., Broch L., Buysse D., Dorsey C., Sateia M. Clinical guideline for the evaluation and management of chronic insomnia in adults. *J Clin Sleep Med.* 2008; 4(5):487–504.

[15] Ohayon M. M. Epidemiology of insomnia: what we know and what we still need to learn. *Sleep Medicine.* 2002; 6(2):97–111.

[16] Seyffert M., Lagisetty P., Landgraf J., Chopra V., Pfeiffer P. N., Conte M. L., Rogers M. A. Internet-Delivered Cognitive Behavioral Therapy to Treat Insomnia: A Systematic Review and Meta-Analysis. *PLoS One.* 2016 Feb 11; 11(2):e0149139. doi: 10.1371/journal.pone.0149139. PMID: 26867139; PMCID: PMC4750912.

[17] National Institute for Health and Care Excellence. NICE guidelines [CG123] *Common mental health disorders: Identification and pathways to care.* May 2011. Available at https://www.nice.org.uk/guidance/cg123/chapter/guidance.

[18] Proudfoot, J., Ryden, C., Everitt, B., Shapiro, D. A., Goldberg, D., Mann, A., & Gray, J. A. (2004). Clinical efficacy of computerised cognitive-behavioural therapy for anxiety and depression in primary care: randomised controlled trial. *The British Journal of Psychiatry*, 185(1), 46-54.

[19] Newby, J. M., Twomey, C., Li, S. S. Y., & Andrews, G. (2016). Transdiagnostic computerised cognitive behavioural therapy for depression and anxiety: a systematic review and meta-analysis. *Journal of Affective Disorders*, 199, 30-41.

[20] Agras, W. S., Fitzsimmons-Craft, E. E., & Wilfley, D. E. (2017). Evolution of cognitive-behavioral therapy for eating disorders. *Behaviour research and therapy*, 88, 26–36. https://doi.org/10.1016/j.brat.2016.09.004.

[21] National Institute for Health and Clinical Excellence and National Collaborating Centre for Mental Health. Depression: Management of depression in primary and secondary care. *NICE*, 2004 (http://www.nice.org.uk/cg023NICEguideline).

[22] Cavanagh K. Turn on, tune in (don't) drop out: engagement, adherence and attrition with internet based mental health interventions. In Bennet-Levy J, et al. *Oxford Guide to Low Intensity Interventions*. Oxford: Oxford University Press, 2010.

[23] Christ C, Schouten MJ, Blankers M, et al. Internet and Computer-Based Cognitive Behavioral Therapy for Anxiety and Depression in Adolescents and Young Adults: Systematic Review and Meta-Analysis. *Journal of Medical Internet Research*. 2020 Sep; 22(9):e17831. doi: 10.2196/17831.

[24] ter Huurne E. D., de Haan H. A., Postel M. G., van der Palen J., Van Der Nagel J. E., De Jong C. A. Web-Based Cognitive Behavioral Therapy for Female Patients With Eating Disorders: Randomized Controlled Trial. *J Med Internet Res*. 2015 Jun 18; 17(6):e152. doi: 10.2196/jmir.3946. PMID: 26088580; PMCID: PMC4526949.

[25] Kurzweil R. (2010, December 28). Technology 25 years hence. *The New York Times*. Retrieved from http://www.nytimes.com/roomfordebate/2010/12/27/why-do-we-need-to-predict-the-future/technology-25-years-hence.

[26] Aardoom, J. J., Dingemans, A. E., Spinhoven, P., & Van Furth, E. F. (2013). Treating eating disorders over the internet: a systematic review and future research directions. *International Journal of Eating Disorders*, 46(6), 539-552.

[27] Hay P., Chinn D., Forbes D., Madden S., Newton R., Sugenor L., ... Ward W. (2014). Royal Australian and New Zealand College of Psychiatrists clinical practice guidelines for the treatment of eating disorders. *Australian and New Zealand Journal of Psychiatry,* 48, 977–1008. doi: 10.1177/0004867414555814.

[28] Sánchez-Ortiz V. C., Munro C., Stahl D., House J., Startup H., Treasure J., ... Schmidt U. (2011). A randomized controlled trial of internet-based cognitive-behavioural therapy for bulimia nervosa or related disorders in a student population. *Psychological Medicine,* 41, 407–417. doi: 10.1017/S0033291710000711.

[29] Wagner G., Penelo E., Wanner C., Gwinner P., Trofaier M., Imgart H., ... Karwautz A. F. K. (2013). Internet-delivered cognitive-behavioural therapy v. conventional guided self-help for bulimia nervosa: Long-term evaluation of a randomised controlled trial. *The British Journal of Psychiatry,* 202, 135–141. doi: 10.1192/bjp.bp. 111.098582.

[30] Aardoom J. J., Dingemans A. E., Spinhoven P., & Van Furth E. F. (2013). Treating eating disorders over the Internet: A systematic review and future research directions. *International Journal of Eating Disorders,* 46, 539–552. doi: 10.1002/eat.22135.

[31] Ackerman, M. J., Filart, R., Burgess, L. P., Lee, I., & Poropatich, R. K. (2010). Developing next-generation telehealth tools and technologies: patients, systems, and data perspectives. *Telemedicine journal and e-health: the official journal of the American Telemedicine Association,* 16(1), 93–95. https://doi.org/10.1089/tmj. 2009.0153.

In: Innovations in Psychiatry ISBN: 978-1-53619-365-7
Editors: Souparno Mitra et al. © 2021 Nova Science Publishers, Inc.

Chapter 6

APPS FOR EATING DISORDERS

Ingrid Haza[*]

BronxCare Health System, Department of Psychiatry
Icahn School of Medicine

ABSTRACT

Mobile apps have significantly evolved since their inception in 1994. This is especially true of mobile apps developed for eating disorders. Whether they aid as an adjunct for therapy or treatment of patients afflicted with eating disorders, these are gaining more traction within the community of providers treating these disorders. Throughout the years different principles have been developed, which have impacted the way patients and providers use said apps. This chapter explores the development of apps, their use, their limitations, and studies available which compare and contrast the pros and cons of apps for eating disorders.

---

[*] Corresponding Author's Email: IHaza@bronxcare.org.

INTRODUCTION

The term eating disorders encompasses a broad range of mental health disorders which include everything from binge eating disorder to anorexia nervosa, with binge eating disorder being the most common. It is believed that these disorders stem from modern- day society's obsession with beauty, having a certain body type, and maintaining a certain level of slimness. Eating disorders are considered very serious and can be fatal. Signs that point to eating disorders include obsessions with body weight, shape, and calorie content. Richard Morton is credited with first describing anorexia nervosa in 1694. As of January 2020, it is reported that approximately 13% of young women and 6% of adults will suffer from a diagnosed eating disorder in their lifetime. This data demonstrates the importance of having access to effective, evidence- based care for this disease. Besides evidence-based therapy for eating disorders, the development of "apps" for mobile devices to aid with treatment for such disorders has been gaining popularity and effectiveness since their development in 2008.

The development of the smart phone, which is a device that has a mobile phone along with computer capabilities, along with rapid growth of multimedia created for smart phones, have paved the way for new opportunities regarding the use of apps on mobile phones for the care of patients. At the end of 2012, mobile device use had reached 91% of the world's population. Studies show that about 74% of the population of the U.S. own mobile smartphones and they are now the most common Internet access device [7].

Apps have been designed for many different purposes and today there are over 1 million apps available and rapidly increasing. It is estimated that one fifth of smart phone users have at least one health related app on their phone. Mental Health and behavioral disorders are the most common type of problem addressed by health apps. Data also demonstrates how only a small proportion of affected individuals seek and receive treatment, partly due to the shame associated with eating disorders, geographical constraints, cost of face-to-face treatment, and the insufficient amounts of trained clinicians available for these evidence- based treatments.

Eating disorder apps have been proposed to support specific components of evidence- based treatments, as well as reduce barriers to treatment access and engagement. It is argued that individuals who suffer from eating disorders must self- monitor frequently as part of their treatment and mobile apps can help provide this component in helping patients self-monitor their behaviors. This concept was tested when a study piloted a weekly text message- based aftercare program for patients who had just received treatment for bulimia on an inpatient unit [7]. The results reported that most patients found this intervention to be "highly convenient, flexible, and well tolerated". Similarly, Shapiro et al. developed and piloted an adjunctive daily SMS based self- monitoring program, for patients receiving 12 weeks of group CBT. Participants in this study were prompted to submit daily information and in return, received automated supportive messages. This initial pilot found an adherence of 87% as well as good acceptability.

DEVELOPMENT OF APPLICATIONS

The U.S. and Australia are leaders in the field of developing online and smartphone or application- based interventions for mental health disorders. This could be attributed to the lack of adequate personnel and the need to provide accessible services for their rural and remote communities. The UK has also set out to promote these types of digital services for treatment of mental health disorders. The UK has commercial organizations that for the most part, have taken the lead on the development of applications for mental health disorders and have produced most of the e-therapies and apps that are currently available. The advantage commercial organizations have over university or academic based institutions when it comes to developing apps, is expertise in online and app- based technology. In house development within the NHS is also promising because they have the ability to use their own trust's internal website development team. This is also more appealing than using commercial companies, as they are more affordable. Projects that have been rolled out by the NHS into clinical services include moderated social network for service users which was first developed for adults with eating disorders called the Support Hope and Recovery Online Network (SHaRON), created in Berkshire Healthcare Foundation Trust. Of note, is the work of Gerhard Andersson et al. in Sweden which is the most important example of e- therapy development within a university setting. The most important aspect of his work is that he and his group were able to obtain their own in- house web developer to create psychological interventions. It is important that developers take into consideration the scalability and sustainability of any digital mental health project, including how the project will be marketed and developed, as this is crucial for it to succeed. One method which can help overcome this barrier, is to work in partnership with a company who can supply digital mental healthcare solutions, and markets the product as well. This would also be key in assuring that the project is able to produce a stable revenue in order to maintain and upgrade the system when needed.

The most important factor to consider when a developing digital mental health app is to have a collaborative team involved in the project. This includes clinicians and researchers who would work with app developers and their company. Having this integrative model allows clinicians and researchers to provide clinical insight and research skills, while the app developers and their companies provide technical knowledge and experience of working with the area of digital healthcare solutions. This effort of co-designing the app would allow for it to engage users, stay relevant, and ensure it is user-friendly. Although there is a promising future in the industry of developing mental health apps and allowing them to be accessible across different populations, it is important to remember that mental health innovation is expanding beyond the pace of scientific evaluation. Therefore, it is imperative to have a framework that ensures the digital era of healthcare is evidence based.

PRINCIPLES BEHIND THE APPS

Data readily available in the International Journal of Eating Disorders demonstrates that out of 800 apps identified that exist for eating disorders at major app stores, only about 39 apps are actually designed for people with eating disorders. Out of those 39 apps, only about 8 of the apps that are relevant for people with eating disorders, had been downloaded more than 5,000 times, which tells us that searching for apps on app stores can be a daunting task with such a small number of apps actually being relevant for patients with eating disorders, compared to the number of apps the search yields. About 5 additional apps had been found for use by eating disorder professionals. Out of the 39 apps for patients with eating disorders, the data reports that the most relevant function of the app was provision of advice, out of 4 major functions identified.

The principles behind the techniques these apps use to help patients with eating disorders includes using technology for computerized cognitive behavioral therapy. These CBT techniques available on the apps, also provide a range of self- help programs for bulimia nervosa and binge eating disorder. In addition to CBT, there are also apps that combine CBT with the guided self-help (GSH) format which combines the use of self-help material with in person visits to complement and help patients implement the treatment intervention. They also include mood rater apps, and digital interventions fully integrated within services. Apps also incorporate readily available informative sections for patients to read about their disorders and be able to get social support they need.

Other technologies that have been studied include the Ecological Momentary Assessment that utilizes ambulatory psychophysiology to measure psychological and physical health constructs in psychiatric disorders. An example are ambulatory measurements of heart rate variability to complement different study designs, which provide insight into psychological and physical health abnormalities concomitant with mental disorders. Heart rate variability has also been used as an outcome measure in both pharmacological and psychosocial treatment trials examining efficacy of interventions in mood, anxiety, and eating disorder symptoms. Considered a transdiagnostic biomarker of autonomic nervous system reactivity, heart rate variability has demonstrated this when results of these studies have been evaluated [8]. It is said that when used in conjunction with ecological momentary assessment, environmental influences, cognition, and emotions, heart rate variability can assess antecedents of mental health symptoms, treatment response and course of symptom presentation.

WAYS PATIENTS AND PROVIDERS USE THE APPS

Application based recording by patients with eating disorders has some benefits including the fact that patients can easily record what they are eating for example. If the goal of the provider is to obtain tracking of psychopathology, apps have an advantage over a written record. Obtaining a patient's record of their food intake, exercise, body weight, which they can conveniently log from their mobile device, can help determine if a person is suffering from an eating disorder. There are also apps for people with eating disorders such as Recovery Record © which allow them to have the ease of communicating with their provider through messages in real time in conjunction with tracking their psychopathology. Having access to a healthcare provider in real time during a crisis can especially be beneficial for the patient, because many of them don't seek the care they need due to the stigma associated with eating disorders. It also allows patients to ease into treatment as they chat through a mobile device, thus reducing the stigma associated with seeking care. Providers can also conveniently track patient's progress by logging in to these apps from a computer or mobile device. Although most of the apps available don't use evidence- based modalities, they can certainly bridge a gap between a patient and access to care, and providers can use such apps as an adjunct to evidence based therapies.

FINDINGS FROM STUDIES

Out of the most popular apps on the market for eating disorders is the app Noom. This app uses cognitive behavioral therapy and guided self-help treatment. A randomized control trial conducted by Hildebrandt et al. tested the efficacy of Noom [5]. Monitor on study retention, adherence, and eating disorder symptoms compared to traditional CBT-GSH. They looked at primary symptom outcomes which included eating disorder examination, objective bulimic episodes, subjective bulimic episodes, and compensatory behaviors. The study describes the utility of CBT-GSH for the treatment of binge eating as desirable because of its properties of scalability or disseminating specialized treatments more widely, evidence of cost effectiveness, and its efficacy among different eating disorder diagnoses. They also emphasize on the importance and priority for mental health conditions such as eating disorders that dissemination and scalability provide. Strengths of the study were described as the fact that they included the use of an active control group, blinded assessments, and detailed assessment of theoretically important mediators and they reported weaknesses of the study as small sample size, and short duration of follow up. However, the study concludes that smartphone apps can in fact improve initial outcomes of CBT-GSH and offer improvement in participant adherence for patients who stay engaged with treatment.

Another paper found in literature review, includes a qualitative study that looks at how apps are used by women with eating disorders [6]. It was reported that as of January 2014, 51.7 percent of the 46 million users who use mobile apps from the health and fitness category were women and that the most popular fitness app during that time was MyFitnessPal. This is an app which allows consumers to track their calories, exercise, and weight. They found that women report their motivation for using such apps to be weight loss even though they may already be at a healthy weight. There are very few research studies when it comes to determining if weight loss apps contribute or exacerbate eating disorders. The authors of the study wanted to see if in fact weight loss apps contributed to eating disorders and they used semi structured interviews on 16 participants who had been diagnosed with an eating disorder and used such apps. Their findings report that there are 2 sides to this argument which are: 1. these apps can in fact exacerbate eating disorders, 2. they can also aid with eating disorder recovery. They also found how weight loss apps can unintentionally promote unhealthy habits or lead to undesired emotions which include how users feel when they manipulate the app to avoid negative emotions. Users reported doing this when they surpassed their daily calorie goal by either exercising more to compensate for their over eating or deciding not to log their intake for that day when they knew they had passed the allotted daily calorie intake. On the other hand, users reported feeling a sense of pride when consuming under the allotted number of calories for the day, which is in contrast to Cordeiro et al. who reported findings that participants did not feel strong positive emotions for eating under their allotted caloric intake for the day. The authors of this study ultimately concluded that their subjects had reported both positive and negative perceptions and effects when using these types of apps and the dynamic nature of weight loss in female users.

A qualitative feedback from user population and clinicians regarding feasibility and acceptance of a smart phone app for treatment of binge eating disorder is another study which aims to conceptualize potential use of an app for eating disorders. The particular app studied, uses self-help material, functions to monitor behavior, and provides in-the-moment interventions. Potential benefits of an app for binge eating disorder also include dissemination beyond just CBT and technological advances in smart phones could improve efficacy of self-help treatments. Capture of real time data is able to be accomplished through Ecological Momentary Assessment, because it uses repeated sampling and is used as a self-monitoring tool. Studies that use EMA along with other forms of technology-based monitoring in individuals with binge eating have reported high levels of compliance and high ease of recording, corroborating that technology-based monitoring is in fact feasible and acceptable method of self- monitoring for this particular population [9].

LIMITATIONS OF THIS TECHNIQUE

The literature also reports that dieting in general poses a risk for developing an eating disorder at some point in a person's life [2]. The exact role for these eating disorder apps is not clearly defined but there is data that reports it can have the potential to trigger, maintain or worsen symptoms of eating disorders. One study reports that 26.1% of participants described that fitness and weight loss apps further perpetuated their disordered eating behaviors and attitudes. Another study that reports similar findings, found that individuals who used their smart phones to track calories endorsed disordered eating and researchers suggested that counting caloric intakes intensified the rigidity that comes with counting calories. Another barrier to this method of using apps on a mobile device, is that it relies solely on what the user is recording whether it be caloric intake, or their exercise for the day and it may not always be reliable. It also lends itself for patients to engage in apps where they obtain unreliable information, feedback, or advice, and may engage in unhealthy or unhelpful communication with other sufferers. Limitations for these apps are also the fact that they aren't capable of analyzing psychopathology and are not always a substitute for the traditional written record. More research needs to be conducted in order to determine the validity and clinical utilities of mobile apps for eating disorders. Therapeutic effects of these apps need further investigations, as very few mental health apps in general have explored this.

It is said that smart phone apps are well suited to disseminate CBT while also addressing many limitations which in person and self-help treatments have for management of binge eating disorder. However, the extent to which smart phone apps are feasible and effective platforms also requires additional study. Previous focus group research has stated that when using self-monitoring apps, consumers prefer prompts and reminders to enter information but also want freedom to set frequency of prompts [9]. There are also concerns about efficacy of Ecological Momentary Intervention regarding the app not being able to accurately assess when an intervention was necessary of helpful [9]. Privacy concerns are also substantially important, given that there is risk of third parties, app developers, and outside companies may have access to identifiable health information. Another great limitation also includes app capabilities to automatically collect location and other data on the user's smartphone.

Future research should focus on examining whether machine learning algorithms can accurately predict instances of behaviors related to eating disorders. It should also focus on the effectiveness and efficacy of smartphone-delivered self- help interventions, as most of the research has been conducted on internet-delivered interventions not designed specifically for smart phones. Further research should also be conducted on investigating how specific components of technology-assisted self-monitoring and interventions can affect outcomes. Also, for future consideration would be providing additional useful services such as maintaining an up-to-date list of the leading eating disorder apps in which their strengths, weaknesses, and potential risks are specified.

Conclusion

Going forward as the need for e-therapies and smart phone apps continues to increase, it is important for interdisciplinary teams to join forces to share information, expertise and experience to develop collaborations. Wearable technology, artificial intelligence, and virtual reality, are all technological advances that open up a wealth of clinical possibilities. The International Society for Research on Internet Interventions is now gaining traction as the stage and platform for such debates. Not only should importance be placed on development of useful apps or technologies, but also importantly on the dissemination of technologies. This is an essential framework to ensure the digital era of healthcare remains evidence based and responsive to the needs of services and service users alike.

REFERENCES

[1] Fairburn, C. & Rothwell, E. (2015). Apps and Eating Disorders: A Systematic Clinical Appraisal. *International Journal of Eating Disorders*, 48, 7, 1038-1046.

[2] Gil, C. (2018). *The Trouble with Tracking*. Duke Center for Eating Disorders. https://eatingdisorders.dukehealth.org/education/trouble-tracking.

[3] Hill, C., et al. (2017). Navigating the challenges of digital health innovation: considerations and solutions in developing online and smartphone-application-based interventions for mental health disorders. *The British Journal of Psychiatry*, 211, 65-69.

[4] Eikey, E. (2016). Privacy and Weight Loss Apps: A First Look at How Women with Eating Disorders Use Social Features. *National Science Foundation*.

[5] Hildebrandt, T., et al. (2017). Randomized Controlled Trial Comparing Smartphone Assisted Versus Traditional Guided Self-Help for Adults with Binge Eating. *International Journal Eating Disorders*, 50(11), 1313-1322.

[6] Eikey, E. & Reddy, M. (2017). "It's Definitely Been a Journey": A Qualitative Study on How Women with Eating Disorders Use Weight Loss Apps. *Self- Tracking Mental Health CHI*, 2017.

[7] Tregarthen, J., et al. (2015). Development of a Smartphone Application for Eating Disorder Self-Monitoring. *International Journal of Eating Disorders*, 48, 7, 972-982.

[8] Juarascio, A., et al. (2015). Perceptions of the feasibility and acceptability of a smartphone application for the treatment of binge eating disorders: Qualitative feedback from a user population and clinicians. *International Jounal Med Inform.*, 84(10), 808-816.

[9] Fairburn, C. Rothwell, E. (2015) Apps and Eating Disorders: A Systematic Clinical Appraisal. *International Journal Eating Disorders*, 48, 1038-1046.

In: Innovations in Psychiatry
Editors: Souparno Mitra et al.
ISBN: 978-1-53619-365-7
© 2021 Nova Science Publishers, Inc.

Chapter 7

PSYCKES AND PDMP

Gurtej Singh Gill*, MD and Sasidhar Gunturu, MD

Department of Psychiatry, BronxCare Health System,
Icahn School of Medicine, Bronx, NY, US

ABSTRACT

This chapter will discuss the importance of Psychiatric Services and Clinical Knowledge Enhancement System (PSYCKES) and Prescription Drug Monitoring Program (PDMP). We will start with the Introduction of PSYCKES and PDMP and will discuss sample cases. Later, we will discuss the practicality of the magnificent clinical database, its limitations, and future direction for utilizing this database for our patients.

INTRODUCTION

An important element of psychiatric evaluation is obtaining collateral. Collateral essentially implies gathering additional information about the

---

* Corresponding Author's Email: GGill@bronxcare.org.

patient from their known contacts apart from history provided by the patient which may give the clinician supplementary information about any previous psychiatric diagnosis and treatment. Collateral can be in the form of information from family members, friends, other providers, medical records, and other available health information systems. Health information systems may be extremely critical, especially when there are patients who do not have any social support systems and may not be able to provide information about past care.

Additionally, controlled substances have been subject to great scrutiny due to the risk of diversion and misuse. Federal laws have established strict tracking mechanisms to account for all controlled substance prescriptions and audit any questionable prescription practices. In this chapter, we discuss a unique health information system from New York State (PSYCKES) and the Federal Prescription Drug Monitoring Program (PDMP).

The Psychiatric Services and Clinical Knowledge Enhancement System (PSYCKES) is an innovative information system for patients enrolled in the New York state Medicaid program. As of 2020, there are over 8 million Medicaid patients who are enrolled in PSYCKES. PSYCKES was developed by a team from the New York State Office of Mental Health (NYSOMH) in partnership with clinical supervisors, clinicians, and information technology staff. This application is secure and HIPAA compliant and access is limited to providers who are involved in direct patient care.

Prescription drug abuse is the leading cause of accidental death in the United States. In 2012, 259 million prescriptions were written for opioid pain relievers, more than one for every US adult. In 2014, 47,055 people died in the United States from a drug overdose, and 61 percent of those deaths were related to opioids. The US opioid epidemic has grown over the last decade and policymakers have suggested a wide variety of strategies to address this crisis.

One policy decision to regulate the prescription of controlled substances has been the use of Prescription Drug Monitoring Programs

(PDMPs). PDMPs are databases that track controlled substance prescriptions from health care providers, usually on a statewide level.

The earliest documented PDMP in the United States (although not termed as such) dates to 1914 when New York State established a short-lived system to track prescriptions of opiates under the Boylan Act. The New York model was the first to require prescribing physicians to submit duplicate prescription forms to a centralized state database. The next state-level PDMP was the "California Triplicate Prescription Program," established in 1939. The rise of the Internet in the 1990s revolutionized the use of PDMPs in the United States from paper-based administrative databases in the early 1900s to modern-day electronic systems that intervene at the point of care.

SAMPLE CASE: TREATMENT AS USUAL

Mr. X is a 44-year-old male with unknown past history who presented to the psychiatric Emergency Department after being brought in by EMS. He is noted to have slurring speech, is responding to internal stimuli, and is extremely agitated. He is unable to provide a history as this is his first visit to this hospital, hence no collateral information or contacts are available. The patient attempts to physically assault a nurse and is prescribed Olanzapine 10 milligram and Lorazepam 4 milligram. Following this, the patient becomes overly sedated and is noted to have shallow breathing.

He had to be immediately transferred to the Medical ED and is ultimately admitted to the ICU.

PART 1: PSYCKES

PSYCKES is a novel tool developed by the Office of Mental Health, New York State. It enables providers to access a patient's comprehensive medical and psychiatric history. The information is presented in both graphical and tabular form.

How does PSYCKES Work?

In order to search for a recipient in PSYCKES, the provider needs either of the following information:

A. Medicaid ID
B. Social security number and/or
C. First name, Last name, and
D. Date of Birth.

PSYCKES gathers information from multiple resources: Administrative data from the Medicaid claims database, billing claims data from managed care plans, prescriptions, laboratories, or other wraparound services.

PSYCKES database provides five years of clinical data that is up to date until approximately 2 weeks prior to the date of review

Additionally, PSYCKES also encompasses data from the following agency

- State Psychiatric center admissions
- AOT provider and contact information (OMH TACT)
- ACT provider and contact information (OMH CAIRS)
- Suicide attempt incidents (OMH NIMRS)
- Managed care plan and HARP status (MC Enrollment Table)
- Health Home enrollment and CM provider information (DOH MAPP)

The data can be accessed without consent in emergency settings. However, access in any other eventuality needs the patient's consent. PSYCKES has some specially protected data, like substance use information and treatment, HIV, Genetic testing, and Obstetrics and Gynecology histories.

PSYCKES contributes to the quality of patient care by informing the rendering provider or care coordinator by flagging clients for quality concerns. Over 60 quality indicators are indicated in PSYCKES which include, e.g., polypharmacy, low medication adherence, general medication health, no diabetes screening when the patient is on Antipsychotics, Acute care utilization (high utilization, readmission). PSYCKES has individual client level reports, Provider level, and statewide reports. It has enhanced quality improvement.

New York State Office of Mental Health (NYSOMH) has a series of interventions aimed at decreasing antipsychotic polypharmacy in New York State Psychiatric hospitals. A study, which was designed as a three-phase intervention, included implementation of the PSYCKES clinical decision making and quality improvement policies. Antipsychotic polypharmacy decreased significantly during phase 1, from 16.9 to 9.7 inpatients per 1,000 and further reduced in phase 2, to 3.9 inpatients per 1,000. In phase 3, the prevalence of antipsychotic polypharmacy remained low at six-month follow-up (3.1inpatients per 1,000).

It is not uncommon for a patient to have had multiple admissions in psychiatric facilities. When a patient is admitted to the Psychiatry emergency or Acute Inpatient Unit, it is necessary to know the patient's medication history, particularly their exposure and response to each medication. Obtaining and reviewing patient records is often a time-consuming and often tricky process. Unfortunately, this information is often not readily available to a clinician at the point of care. PSYCKES facilitates access to aggregated patient data and has a Clinical Summary organized by sections for a rapid review, like an EMR.

The data summarized in PSYCKES include:

- General Information
- Current Care Coordination
- Alerts and Incidents
- Quality Flags
- Plans and Documents

- Screenings and Assessments
- Diagnoses
- Care Coordination History
- Medications
- Outpatient Services
- Hospital/ER Services
- Living Support/Residential
- Laboratory and Radiology
- Dental, Vision, Medical Equipment, Transportation

Limitations of PSYCKES

PSYCKES data can provide important information about treatment history but may not represent an entire clinical picture. Thus, there is still a need for improvement in PSYCKES. Some of the limitations in PSYCKES are as follows:

- PSYCKES covers only Medicaid patients, and if it can cover other insurances, there will be more diversity in the database we get from PSYCKES.
- PSYCKES covers only the past five years of data. Many patients have a very long psychiatric history; data covering more than five years would benefit our patient population.
- If we incorporate PSYCKES in our hospital based EMR, PSYCKES would be more user friendly and much more easily accessible.
- Accuracy is dependent on coding and billing and data elements are limited to the claims that filed.
- There is a time lag between services rendered and billed. This may bring about some gap in terms of time that is lost in uploading the data.
- Client data affected by hospitalizations, loss of Medicaid coverage.

- PSYCKES data can provide important information about treatment history but may not represent an entire clinical picture.
- Self-reported data may appear inconsistent.

PART 2: PRESCRIPTION DRUG MONITORING PROGRAM

The introduction of a prescription drug monitoring program dates to efforts to control non-medical use and/or medical abuse of prescription drugs, particularly prescription opioids and benzodiazepines. It is a preventative program that aims to safeguard the supply of both legal and illicit prescription medications.

How Does PDMP Work

PDMPs are now in use in 49 states, the District of Columbia, Guam, and Puerto Rico. Missouri is now the only state without a statewide PDMP, although the city of St. Louis operates one. PDMPs require retail pharmacists to enter data from prescriptions for controlled substances into a centralized electronic database. This data identifies the prescriber, dispenser, and patient, as well as the drug, dose, and amount dispensed. Some PDMPs require additional information that helps pharmacists/prescribers track and identify duplicates and stolen forms.

For data to be accurate, the name and date of birth must be reported factually by the patient, written correctly on the prescription, entered without error by the pharmacy, and lastly entered precisely by the clinician searching for the report. The purpose of the PDMP is to detect and reduce diversion, abuse, and misuse of prescription medications classified as controlled substances and to reduce associated harms. Some of the benefits of PDMP are as follows:

1. Pain is a condition that is almost impossible to measure. It is difficult to differentiate a patient who legitimately suffers pain from one who is presenting with pain for secondary gain. The PDMP system may help identify persons who have no genuine medical need. Thus, it can add accuracy to providers' clinical judgments to determine the requirements for pain management by reviewing patients' past prescription history. A real-time PDMP may help alleviate over-provision and potential diversion of these pharmaceuticals. As an added benefit, prescribers may monitor the database to detect forged prescriptions or stolen prescription pads.
2. PDMPs can help identify any suspected fraudulent prescribing or illegal activities related to the dispensing of controlled substances. For Example, In Florida, PDMP played an important role in the improvements of the prescription drug-abuse record. In 2010, among the top 100 oxycodone prescribing physicians in the nation 90 were in Florida. This number dropped to only 13 in 2011.
3. PDMP has the most up-to-date, real-time information about controlled substance use across all practices, and physician's access to that information can support clinical judgment and improve the quality of care. PDMP can help identify patients who are receiving multiple legitimate prescriptions but are at risk of complications from polypharmacy. It is more comfortable checking a PDMP report than mandating urine drug screening, which can result in disruption of the patient-physician relationship. The awareness among patients about the PDMP database would enhance the patient-provider relationship.
4. PDMP may help identify those at the highest risk for opioid overdose and create an opportunity for intervention when aberrant behavior is first noted. A survey in Maine, USA found PDMP helped over a third of the prescribers referring their patients to substance abuse treatment.
5. Real-time access to a patient's prescription history increases the prescriber's confidence in prescribing. For instance, a study of real-time PDMP in an emergency department in Ohio found that

after reviewing the patient's prescription history clinicians changed their opioid prescription in 41% of cases, of which more than a third (39%) received higher doses than initially planned.
6. Data from PDMP can also be used to identify geographic areas with high rates of opioid misuse, reveal changes in prescribing practices and patterns, and spatial information in a small geographical area allowing the introduction of focused interventions in those communities.

Limitations of PDMP

Some physicians, for valid reasons, may be relatively high prescribers. PDMP may flag them to be inappropriate prescribers. While most physicians would be expected to support interventions to prevent fraudulent prescribing, criminal prosecutions of physicians prescribing large amounts of opioids could make the physicians reluctant to prescribe controlled substances for fear of legal retribution which is also called the "chilling effect." The chilling effect could also lead to increased prescribing of alternate medications which is also known as the substitution effect, even if they are inferior in terms of efficacy or have greater side effects.

1. Patients can be falsely labeled as "pseudo-addicts." Patients enrolled in PDMP may deter legitimate prescribing for a patient with a history of receiving pain medication from several physicians. Such patients may be "pseudo-addicts" whose pain has not been controlled by sub-therapeutic analgesics doses and who is genuinely seeking relief of pain, and not to support an addiction.
2. Like prescribers, patients may fear coming under scrutiny from law-enforcement if they use medications monitored by the PDMP. Patients worry about the additional cost of more frequent office visits if prescribers become more cautious about writing prescriptions with refills. Patients may feel embarrassed or

abandoned when questioned about substance use and then excluded from an expected treatment. Patients with a history of opioid dependence may not receive treatment for valid conditions. This can result in people not returning to the physicians for on-going care and refusal can eventually push some patients into the illicit market. For instance, the opioid use crackdown in Florida was followed by increased use of heroin and resulted in increased overdose presentations in the emergency department (4). CDC data show a decrease in opioid analgesic overdose in 2012, but also show a 35% increase in heroin deaths over the same year and a continued rise in drug overdose deaths overall.

3. PDMPs may wrongfully suspect and categorize some physicians as fraudulent prescribers when they are prescribing in good faith but lack training in identifying prescription drug abuse or recognize the warning signs of drug diversion. In the USA over 40% of primary care physicians report difficulty in discussing the possibility of prescription medication abuse with patients and over 90% fail to detect symptoms of substance abuse.

4. There is discomfort among physicians and patients that PDMP means that a medical consultation is no longer a private affair, and raises concerns about maintaining patient/provider privacy, confidentiality, and data security. Privacy concerns may also cause some patients to avoid or to postpone needed medication for fear of being labeled as drug addicts.

5. Recognition of prescription drug abuse has evoked many regulatory and legislative actions, and, in some settings, healthcare policy is increasingly influenced by law-enforcement agencies. By nature, law-enforcement agencies will focus on the abuse side of the equation, without always considering any detrimental effect from inadequate prescribing. In some settings, with origins in law-enforcement, PDMPs are now seen as a tool of the police rather than an important component of patient safety.

6. PDMP can create additional time constraints for physicians. Identification of potential abuse warrants a series of responses

including counseling and referral for substance abuse treatment, which are time-consuming. These pressures, encouraging physicians to use PDMP databases in settings that are voluntary has been a challenge: a part of which relates to making the databases more convenient for physicians that include real-time data provision, easy recovery of forgotten passwords, and easy navigation to the web portal.

SAMPLE CASE: TREATMENT WITH THE ACCESS TO PSYCKES AND PDMP

Mr. X presents to the ED with a similar presentation. On review of PSYCKES and PDMP, it is noted that the patient has multiple Substance Use treatment admissions for Opioid and Benzodiazepine Use Disorder. He was recently discharged on Methadone and Klonopin. Noting this history, the possibility of concurrent benzodiazepine and methadone overdose is considered. The patient is restrained and Narcan is administered, with gradual restoration of lucidity.

DISCUSSION AND FUTURE DIRECTIONS FOR PSYCKES AND PDMP

In today's practice of psychiatry, PSYCKES plays an integral role as it provides a comprehensive patient's history in no time. The data is updated regularly, and it helps the physician reach a comprehensive clinical decision and prescribe medications with the help of data that is readily available in PSYCKES. Today, we have PSYCKES available very readily and can access patients' records if we have access to the internet. The most significant advantage is that it is HIPAA compliant and secure health data. We see some significant improvements in PSYCKES regularly. There are some new releases in PSYCKES 6.7.0, some of which include:

- Enhancements to Consent: PSYCKES, BHCC, and DOH Adult Health Home
- Bulk Population Management Advanced Views in Recipient Search Results Page
- New Alert: Concurrent Opioid-Benzodiazepine
- Opioid Medications & Controlled Substances Filters
- Children's Waiver Status
- Any OMH Outpatient Specialty MH Services Population Filter

PDMP has shown promise but has limitations and needs work to improve for maximum effectiveness. If PDMPs are to be successful, further improvements are needed in terms of accuracy, accessibility, and interpretability of the data. Some of the suggestive improvements can be following

1. Easy and limited efforts to access to the program on the part of the clinician is essential for increased use.
2. To maximize the use of the PDMP, we need additional research to determine how this program can be used in the clinical setting to identify the upper limit of the value that red flags in a PDMP report which may require urgent intervention from the clinician.
3. Improved patient education for those receiving opioids is needed to fully explain the risks and benefits of opioids and other controlled medications.
4. Training clinicians in chronic pain management and responsible opioid prescribing may do more to reduce opioid prescribing than access to PDMP.
5. Patients determined to deceive the system may do so by crossing state borders in states without effective data sharing or reporting false personal information when registering with hospitals and clinics. The promise of PDMPs is to improve data sharing among providers in order to avert diversion and prescribing to those at risk of abuse and overdose. However, this data sharing is limited to

a few data points. PDMPs could provide means of communication between providers within an Internet portal that is compliant with privacy laws and allows better communication on controlled medications. This would also allow emergency providers to notify other prescribers of patients who have either overdosed or are at risk for overdose.

REFERENCES

[1] Office of Mental Health, New York State. *PSYCKES*. New York State Department of Health. https://omh.ny.gov/omhweb/psyckes_medicaid/about/.

[2] Cohen, T., Kaufman, D., White, T., Segal, G., Staub, A. B., Patel, V. L., & Finnerty, M. T. (2004, January). Cognitive evaluation of an innovative psychiatric clinical knowledge enhancement system. In *Medinfo* (pp. 1295-1299).

[3] Finnerty, M. T., Kealey, E., Leckman-Westin, E., Gupta, N., White, T. M., Engel, G. M., & Opler, L. A. (2011). Best practices: Long-term impact of web-based tools, leadership feedback, and policies on inpatient antipsychotic polypharmacy. *Psychiatric Services*, 62(10), 1124-1126.

[4] Griggs, C. A., Weiner, S. G., & Feldman, J. A. (2015). Prescription drug monitoring programs: examining limitations and future approaches. *Western Journal of Emergency Medicine*, 16(1), 67.

[5] Holmgren, A. J., Botelho, A., & Brandt, A. M. (2020). A History of Prescription Drug Monitoring Programs in the United States: Political Appeal and Public Health Efficacy. *American journal of public health*, 110(8), 1191-1197.

[6] Patrick, S. W., Fry, C. E., Jones, T. F., & Buntin, M. B. (2016). Implementation of prescription drug monitoring programs associated with reductions in opioid-related death rates. *Health Affairs*, 35(7), 1324-1332.

[7] Islam, M. M., & McRae, I. S. (2014). An inevitable wave of prescription drug monitoring programs in the context of prescription opioids: pros, cons and tensions. *BMC pharmacology and toxicology*, 15(1), 46.

In: Innovations in Psychiatry
Editors: Souparno Mitra et al.

ISBN: 978-1-53619-365-7
© 2021 Nova Science Publishers, Inc.

Chapter 8

ECOLOGICAL MOMENTARY ASSESSMENT (EMA)

Souparno Mitra[*], *MD*
BronxCare Health System Department of Psychiatry,
Icahn School of Medicine, Bronx, NY, US

ABSTRACT

In this chapter, we discuss the importance of Ecological Momentary Assessment. We start with a description of what Ecological Momentary Assessment is and move on to discuss its applications as it relates to clinical work and research as well as the advantages and disadvantages of this methodology. We also review papers which have looked into the efficacy of this intervention and discuss the future of this methodology.

INTRODUCTION

Psychiatry relies greatly on subjective assessments of an individual's current mental state. Be it their mood, delusions or cognitions, there may

---

[*] Corresponding Author's Email: SMitra@bronxcare.org.

be variability in responses relating to their perception about a certain situation based on whether the response is immediate or remote. Time, they say, is a great healer. Time also gives an individual the opportunity to reflect, ponder and rationalize their responses to certain circumstances.

This poses a challenge to provision of mental health services in an outpatient setting. In this setting, the provider meets with the client at regularly scheduled intervals which may be once a week or even once a month. Now, whether the client remembers how they felt a week before their visit or yesterday is a question that is completely dependent on the client's memory and ability to suppress or repress unwanted thoughts and cognition.

We will discuss this chapter's topic with a sample case which we shall review first with the Treatment as Usual (TAU) Model, which involves regularly scheduled outpatient appointments. Subsequently, we will introduce and discuss Ecological Momentary Assessment (EMA) and its theories and principles as well as findings from studies on this assessment tool. We will then close the loop by reviewing the same case with the application of EMA in the provision of care to the client.

Sample Case: Treatment as Usual

Ms. M is a 35-year-old female with past history of Generalized Anxiety Disorder and Cocaine Use Disorder. She is domiciled in her own apartment, works as an investment banker and is married with 3 children. She works at a firm on Wall Street and works from 9 am to 8 pm Monday to Friday and spends her weekends with her children and family and also socializing with her friends.

She has been suffering from anxiety since the age of 16. Her anxiety started in high school prior to her SATs and gradually increased to debilitating levels. When she entered college, she tried to suppress her anxiety with substances such as alcohol and cocaine. She drinks socially at present, drinking 1-2 drinks approximately every 1-2 weeks. However, her cocaine use has become problematic with her use increasing to approximately 5-6 lines every day. Her cocaine use began recreationally in college and increased to daily use during her first year as a financial analyst in her firm. She would spend a large portion of her paycheck on drugs and would often use cocaine in between her work hours.

When she realized her use was reaching problematic proportions, she sought inpatient treatment at a rehab where she was managed with motivational and psychodynamic therapy and subsequently, she transitioned to outpatient care at a dual-diagnosis clinic. Currently, she meets her psychiatrist for an hour every month for medication management with an antidepressant and her therapist two times a month for hour long sessions in between her work hours.

She finds it difficult to find time given her busy work and social schedule and has often enquired with her care team about the possibility of remote therapy sessions. When her therapist assesses her about her current stressors and triggers for craving of cocaine, she has trouble remembering and explaining certain situations that may have led to such cravings. This has led to brief periods of relapse and periods of self-doubt, exacerbation of anxiety and disruptions in her inter-personal relationships.

Her therapist also wishes that there was a therapeutic tool which would enable real time assessment of her triggers and symptoms and offer brief interventions.

WHAT IS ECOLOGICAL MOMENTARY ASSESSMENT (EMA)

Ecological Momentary Assessments are assessment methodologies which utilize real-time assessment of symptomatology, triggers and relations to others multiple times in a day. This data is collected via electronic methods such as smartphones, tablets or smartwatches while the subjects are in their natural environments, going about their lives. We should consider EMA as an electronic diary, where the subject enters observations when alerts are sent several times a day.

EMA is not a single methodology but a combination of different discrete methodologies (Schiffman, 2008). It was developed in response to the limitations caused by self-reports and physician data. This included recall bias, and inter-evaluator discrepancies. The term was coined in 1994 by Stone and Schiffman. A study, (Schiffman 2008), carried out a comprehensive literature search and discovered almost 3000 articles on the topic. Stone et al. (2007b), Hektner et al. (2007), and Fahrenberg & Myrtek (2001) have written books on EMA and its applications.

Some common methodologies used for assessments using EMA include interpersonal interaction diaries (Reis & Wheeler 1991), ambulatory physiological monitoring (Kop et al. 2001), and collection of medication compliance data by instrumented pill bottles (Byerly et al. 2005).

One of the core principles of EMA includes the collection of data repeatedly, in the subject's natural environment and as close to real-time as possible. One of the aims of EMA is to give researchers a common structural framework which encompasses different research methodologies and apply them to their studies on physical and psychological methodologies.

How Does EMA Work

EMA had been developed to mitigate the effects of recall bias and the dependence on the patient's remote and recent memory. When a patient signs up for a research protocol or treatment modality that involves EMA, the following steps are generally followed:

- Patient visits the office and the procedures involved in EMA as well as what the expectations are explained to the patient. They

- sign a HIPAA consent and also provide contact information which may include a phone number or email address.
- They are trained about this assessment method and are provided with practice lessons and devices that may be needed to participate in this assessment form.
- Depending on their preferred mode of communication, an email or text message is sent to the patient daily, or at scheduled intervals with a link
- When patient's open the link it guides them to various assessment tools such as mood or anxiety scales where they self-report their perceived emotions at the time.
- They can also journal or note particular incidents or stressors that they experienced since the last assessment which may have exacerbated their illness.
- Along with this, certain e-therapy techniques such as resilience-building exercises, or meditation and mindfulness can be attached for the patient to improve their coping skills.
- The frequency of assessments is decided collaboratively by the provider and the patient depending on their illness and the severity of their illness and goals of the assessment.
- Following these assessments, patients' meet with their providers and can discuss and develop new treatment plans based on the results of the assessment.

APPLICATIONS OF EMA

EMA has found application in:

- Suicide Risk Assessment
- Non-Suicidal Self Injurious Behavior
- Substance Use research to assess for cravings, triggers and relapses
- Depression: to identify stressors, monitor activity, mood and sleep

- Anxiety Disorders: To monitor stressors, severity of illness, sleep and physiological symptoms
- Psychotic Disorders: To monitor symptomatology, stressors and functionality
- Eating Disorders
- ADHD
- Heart Rate Variability
- Autism Spectrum Disorders
- Juvenile Idiopathic Arthritis
- Mobile EKG and EEGs
- Provision of e-therapy modalities.
- Borderline Personality Disorders

FINDINGS FROM REVIEW OF LITERATURE

A comprehensive literature search was done on PubMED and led to the following results:

Ecological Momentary Assessment Is a Neglected Methodology in Suicidology (Davidson et al. 2016)

This paper looked at the use of EMA in the assessment of suicidality. It looks at materials used such as paper journals, Personal Digital Assistants (PDAs) and cellphones. It talks of the importance of this method in the theoretical conception of suicide, and the implications for suicide risk assessments.

The paper talks of flaws in paper journals such as missed schedule times as they depend on alarms set on watches. Secondly, there is no way to verify when the journal was completed. A solution to the second issue was the inclusion of an electronic timestamp in the journal which recorded the time it was opened. Other issues found were employing branching logic, the burden associated with carrying a binder and data security, especially if there was a loss or theft.

PDAs permit for flexible assessment protocols, allowing branching logics and allowing real time automated responses and time-stamping. PDAs have been largely replaced with smartphones. Also, participants may not remember to carry these devices. A matter extremely important for suicide research is that real-time access to participants is not available on some devices.

At present, however, with the advent of smartphones, PDAs and paper journals have been replaced by smartphones. The possibility of real time responses is a boon for providers as automated emails may be set up to alert staff about concerning responses.

The paper also talks of the two sampling schemes: Event based sampling and time-based sampling. Event based sampling asks participants to respond to questions each time they experience a behavior. Time based sampling asks for responses at set periods of time. Event-based sampling requires participants to recognize the pre-determined behavior while time-based sampling should ask questions especially about how they felt since their last assessment. The assessment period is especially important for self-directed violent behavior.

The paper reviewed 8 papers studying EMA for suicidality. One of the papers, Links et al. 2007 assessed 27 mood states and Scale for Suicidal Ideation and Suicide Behavior Questionnaire. Results showed that negative mood intensity related to suicidal ideation and behavior. The second paper was by the same authors in 2008 wherein they studied the relationship between affective instability and suicidal behavior in patients with Borderline Personality Disorder. Results showed that patient with high negative mood intensity and mood amplitude had higher SBQ scores. Another study (Nisenbaum et al. 2010), investigated negative mood variability in patients with BPD. It showed there was no significant mood variability diurnally and between participants and was impacted by suicidal ideation, hopelessness and depression. Nock et al. 2009, assessed suicidal and non-suicidal behavior in adolescents. It showed participants experiencing SI once a week and no suicide attempts. Episodes of NSSI were preceded by NSSI thoughts that were more intense and shorter duration with feeling of rejection, numbness, self-hatred and anger. NSSI also served an intrapersonal reinforcement function and helped regulate affect and cognition. Muhlenkamp et al. 2009 studied positive and negative affect before and after NSSI in women with Bulimia. They found that positive affect tended to be lower and negative affect higher prior to NSSI and that positive affect increased after NSSI. Another study using the same dataset found that high trait affective lability and history of suicide attempts predict NSSI. Palmier-Claus et al. 2012 studied relationship between positive and negative affective instability and suicidal thoughts in 27 individuals who were thought to be "ultra-high risk" for psychosis. Results showed that variability of positive and negative affect predicted the frequency of suicidal ideation and negative affect variability predicted the severity of suicidal ideation. Humber, 2013, studied anger and NSSI and suicidal ideation in incarcerated male inmates. Results revealed that anger was related to NSSI but not to suicidal ideation.

The benefits discussed in the paper include lesser bias than retrospective reports, a nuanced view of variable over time. This modality also allows testing certain theories of suicidal behavior such as Fluid Vulnerability Report which holds that all individuals have a baseline suicidal risk. It can also study temporal variations and impacts of other risk factors. The correlation of substance use can also be studied using this modality. They also talk of sending out reminder messages to remind patients to have a look at safety plans and monitor own behavior.

Ecological Momentary Assessment and Intervention in the Treatment of Psychotic Disorders: A Systematic Review (Bell et al. 2017)

This paper talks of the applications of EMA in treatment of psychotic disorders and is a review of current literature. The paper talks of how EMA is used to research mechanisms of underlying symptoms. The authors used a PRISMA model for comprehensive literature review. They identified 1623 studies and 78 were evaluated in detail and 9 were included for the review.

Four studies looked at warning signs of symptom relapse using an intervention called Information Technology-Aided Relapse Prevention Program in Schizophrenia. Patients and caregivers were asked to complete the Early Warning Signs Questionnaire, the responses were monitored by the treatment team. The adherence to monitoring protocols were low (39%). The studies showed reduction in hospital events and total hospital days.

Five of the studies looked at psychosocial functioning. The app-based FOCUS and SMS delivered Mobile Assessment and Intervention for Schizophrenia were used on a daily basis. They provided medication reminders and momentary interventions for challenging cognition, coping and promotion of healthy behaviors.

Three studies looked at compensation for cognitive difficulties and promotion of activities of daily living and goal achievements (appointments, medication compliance and inhibiting undesirable behavior).

Dropout rated for all studies was found to be 15% (0%-36%). Reasons included loss of device, illness severity, loss of interest and intervention nonengagement. Mean response rates were 80%. The paper found that EMA can be used for illness self-management, and improving activities of daily living.

Ecological Momentary Interventions for Depression and Anxiety (Schueller et al. 2017)

This paper looks at the utility of EMA for Depression and Anxiety. It provides mechanisms, study designs and therapeutic measures that can be incorporated for design of an EMA for depression and anxiety.

EMAs intended to reduce depression should do so via interventions aimed at outcomes such as engagement in pleasurable activities and increasing positive emotions. They also found use of therapeutic measures such as acceptance and commitment therapy and interpersonal therapy, though the majority utilized Cognitive-Behavioral Therapy, Behavioral Activation, relaxation and self-monitoring. A recent meta-analysis found 33 studies targeting symptoms of depression, as well as anxiety, perceived stress and positive psychological functioning. EMA was found to have small to medium effect on within person change. The effect size was more with support systems in place. EMAs were found to be more effective when they complement and extend treatment as usual. They can increase homework adherence and reinforce therapeutic concepts in real-world settings.

For anxiety, the paper found a lot of similarities with EMIs for depression. They had similar diversity of concept and efficacy. 15 studies found an effect size of 0.47 which was similar to that for depression. 7 studies found a decrease of generalized anxiety by an effect size of 0.32. EMA which target stress were superior to controls. Only two studies used automated sensors.

The paper recommends the use of microrandomized trials to assess efficacy of EMAs. Advances in analytics such as data mining and machine learning can help understand EMA at an individual level.

From Ecological Momentary Assessment (EMA) to Ecological Momentary Intervention (EMI): Past and Future Directions for Ambulatory Assessment and Interventions in Eating Disorders (Smith et al. 2019)

This paper talks of the utility of EMA in the assessment of eating disorders, by looking at the realms of type, frequency and temporal sequencing of ED Symptoms in natural environment.

The paper found that for ambulatory assessments using EMA there has been an expansion of constructs that are being assessed. They also found that there is greater level of exploration of the state vs trait processes, integration of objective and passive approaches and consideration of methodological issues. The paper found recent research focusing mostly on Mobile Health technologies with minimal EMA Components. There are many areas that may be exciting for research and include: Integration of passive data collection, using EMA in treatment evaluation and design, evaluating dynamic processes, including diverse samples and developing and evaluating adaptive tailored EMAs.

This paper thus provided some future directions of research in the field of eating disorders.

Using Mobile-Technology-Based Ecological Momentary Assessment (EMA) Methods with Youth: A Systematic Review and Recommendations (Heron et al. 2017)

This paper describes the use of EMA for child and adolescent patients. It focuses on mobile based utilization. It talks of EMA providing reduced. retrospective recall and associated biases. These biases are even more important in children. With this modality, children and adolescents may have improved reporting of pain, treatment adherence, sleep and disease symptoms. It will also enable data collection in settings children are exposed to, such as in school or at home.

The data collection methods seen in the data search had a duration range of 4 to 31 days, though one study had one of 120 days. One study, which collected data from a substance use treatment program, had a one month on, one month off data collection schedule. This schedule is described as a measurement burst design. Most studies included participants for 4-5 days as a burst and later for 8-25 days. The studies asked for assessments from participants at random times of the day. The daily frequency ranged from 2 to 9 times a day, the average being 4.4 times a day. In a few studies, participants were asked to initiate assessments after eating or a particular interaction (event-contingent sampling)

The two most common hardware used were smartphones and mobile phones, while two studies used the iPod Touch. The studies used mobile apps, text messages, phone calls using interactive voice response to answer assessments.

Some of the factors mentioned considerations such as logistical issues including loss or malfunctioning of hardware or poor reception. Two-thirds of the studies reported adaptations made to EMA hardware or content to make them user friendly. One of the major considerations was to understand how to manage responses during school hours. Some measures included schedules which avoided class hours or obtaining teacher's approval.

71% of studies trained the participants and only 44% of the studies reported completion rates; of the studies that did, the average survey completion rate was 76%. Some of the disorders for which EMA was used included affective disorders, autism spectrum disorders, substance use disorders, juvenile idiopathic arthritis, asthma, binge eating disorders, attention-deficit hyperactivity disorder, diabetes, borderline personality disorder, anxiety.

This paper showed the wide range of illnesses that can be addressed with the help of EMA and the modalities that may be used for the same.

A Comprehensive Review of Psychophysiological Applications for Ecological Momentary Assessment in Psychiatric Populations (Raugh et al. 2019)

This paper talks of the use of EMA for psychophysiological assessments. It reviews utility of EMA for EKG, Blood pressure, EEG, electrooculography, electromyography and others. The advantages of mobile monitoring include ecological validity, temporal precision and concurrent evaluation of internally and externally generated contexts. Disadvantages mentioned include loss of experimental control and the difficulty of conducting such studies.

Psychophysiological assessment involves assessing the autonomic and central nervous system during a psychological process such as cognitive ability and affective processing.

The paper goes on to describe the utility of EMA for each measurement modality. They found 76 papers looking at EKG readings such as Heart rate, Heart rate variability, additional Heart rate (marker of sympathetic activity). These reading can be used for panic attack, phobia, hallucinations or binges.

Blood pressure is the second modality mentioned. They found 23 studies focused on blood pressure. These pressures showed associations with hostility, pessimism, emotional responsivity, negative mood, anxiety, panic and negative social interactions.

Respiration was another modality mentioned which used plethysmegraphy and transcutaneous sensors. This can be used for ambulatory feedback and therapeutic measures. This has found application in anxiety and panic disorders.

Electrodermal activity or skin conductance was also used to determine sweat gland activation during arousal. It helps in determining physiological and emotional arousal. This again found application in panic states. EEG was studied for PTSD, Borderline Personality Disorders, psychotic disorders and sleep studies. Some studies used combined measures such as pulse and temperature or temperature, activity and voice analysis.

The advantages mentioned including bypassing the problems with self-report, passive collection of data.

SAMPLE CASE: EMA

Ms M's Therapist through her review of protocols encounters EMA and discusses the option of incorporating this modality in her treatment. Ms M agrees with the plan. They incorporate mobile app based EMA which carries out twice a day random and contingency based assessment of her triggers and cravings for substance use and also her symptoms of anxiety. Depending on the assessment the app then carries out virtual therapy protocols such as contingency management, meditation and biofeedback. In case of severe scores, it alerts her therapist and also provides crisis resources.

Ms M has a response rate of 80% at the time of her first visit after starting EMA. The assessment tools have provided her with real time data about the possible triggers for her cocaine cravings and use as well as for her anxiety symptoms. She has been able to identify arguments with her husband or talk about "partying" at work to be triggers for her substance use. With the help of the virtual contingency management measures, she has been able to reduce the frequency and amount of her cocaine use. She has also identified lack of a structured routine as one of the triggers for her anxiety and with the help of therapeutic measures through EMA has been able to work on structuring her day further.

Ms M after 4 months showed a period of abstinence from Cocaine as well as reduced Beck's Anxiety Inventory scores. She has been experiencing improved psychosocial functioning and has been able to cope with her daily work schedules. She is adherent with her treatment and follow up and has been having a more "wholesome" experience.

ADVANTAGES AND DISADVANTAGES OF EMA

Advantages:

- Avoids recall bias
- Can provide real-time assessments
- Not dependent on respondent's bias
- Can permit immediate interventions
- Allows remote alert for providers
- Can be used for research as well as therapeutic measures

Disadvantages:

- Equipment and technology dependent
- Depends on network connectivity
- Risk of attrition
- Necessity for detailed study modeling
- Not enough literature that investigates the benefits of the methods
- Requires motivation on the part of the patient to respond and participate on a regular basis
- Risk of redundancy

CONCLUSION

EMA, thus far, has been a successful research modality. Studies have shown it to be beneficial for real time assessment for disorders such as anxiety and substance use. There is definite scope for improvement in a more structured model for assessment and intervention as well as the improvement of technology that may be used, especially in underserved communities.

Further research focusing on the appropriate frequency and duration of EMA as well as the content of assessment may improve compliance as well as lead to more effective and user-friendly therapeutic results.

REFERENCES

Bell, I. H., Lim, M. H., Rossell, S. L., & Thomas, N. (2017). Ecological Momentary Assessment and Intervention in the Treatment of Psychotic Disorders: A Systematic Review. *Psychiatric services* (Washington, D.C.), 68(11), 1172–1181. https://doi.org/10.1176/appi.ps.201600523.

Bertz, J. W., Epstein, D. H., & Preston, K. L. (2018). Combining ecological momentary assessment with objective, ambulatory measures of behavior and physiology in substance-use research. *Addictive behaviors*, 83, 5–17. https://doi.org/10.1016/j.addbeh.2017.11.027.

Collin L. Davidson, Michael D. Anestis & Peter M. Gutierrez (2017) Ecological Momentary Assessment is a Neglected Methodology in Suicidology, *Archives of Suicide Research,* 21:1, 1-11, doi: 10.1080/13811118.2015.1004482.

Heron, K. E., Everhart, R. S., McHale, S. M., & Smyth, J. M. (2017). Using Mobile-Technology-Based Ecological Momentary Assessment (EMA) Methods with Youth: A Systematic Review and Recommendations. *Journal of pediatric psychology*, 42(10), 1087–1107. https://doi.org/10.1093/jpepsy/jsx078.

Moskowitz, D. S., & Young, S. N. (2006). Ecological momentary assessment: what it is and why it is a method of the future in clinical psychopharmacology. *Journal of psychiatry & neuroscience: JPN*, 31(1), 13–20.

Raugh IM, Chapman HC, Bartolomeo LA, Gonzalez C, Strauss GP. A comprehensive review of psychophysiological applications for *ecological momentary assessment in psychiatric populations. Psychol Assess.* 2019; 31(3):304-317. doi: 10.1037/pas0000651.

Schueller, S. M., Aguilera, A., & Mohr, D. C. (2017). Ecological momentary interventions for depression and anxiety. *Depression and anxiety*, 34(6), 540–545. https://doi.org/10.1002/da.22649.

Shiffman, S., Stone, A. A., Hufford, M. R. (2008). Ecological Momentary Assessment. *Annual Review of Clinical Psychology*, 4, 132. https://doiorg.eresources.mssm.edu/10.1146/annurev.clinpsy.3.022806.091415.

Smith, K. E., & Juarascio, A. (2019). From Ecological Momentary Assessment (EMA) to Ecological Momentary Intervention (EMI): Past and Future Directions for Ambulatory Assessment and Interventions in Eating Disorders. *Current psychiatry reports*, 21(7), 53. https://doi.org/10.1007/s11920-019-1046-8.

In: Innovations in Psychiatry
Editors: Souparno Mitra et al.
ISBN: 978-1-53619-365-7
© 2021 Nova Science Publishers, Inc.

Chapter 9

APPS FOR CHILD AND ADOLESCENT MENTAL HEALTH DISORDERS

Himansh Saxena[*], MD

BronxCare Health System, Department of Psychiatry,
Icahn School of Medicine, Bronx, NY, US

ABSTRACT

This chapter has a brief description of the various mental illnesses and the free online resources that are available to administer children. The importance of having free online resources at the disposal of parents or caregivers to administer in the time of uncertainty is of paramount. Having access to free online applications with a push or a click of a button on their cell phone or a computer can help caregivers with children to seek proper care for the child. It is by far one of the most essential tools a caregiver should have in their arsenal when dealing with various mental illnesses that stricken children at various age groups. These online tools can educate and direct a parent, a guardian, a teacher, a babysitter or any adult taking care of a child to seek physician's care if needed.

---

[*] Corresponding Author's Email: HSaxena@bronxcare.org.

INTRODUCTION

Online screening tools have become one of the easiest and quickest ways for teachers, guardians, and other care takers to ascertain whether a child or an adolescent is experiencing a mental illness and requires further evaluation by a healthcare provider.

Use of these tools help detect and identify children at risk and prevent critical outcomes.

MENTAL ILLNESS IN THE CHILD AND ADOLESCENT POPULATION

Neurodevelopment Disorders

Intellectual Disability: Onset during the developmental period that includes both intellectual and adaptive functioning deficits.

Communication Disorders: Onset during the developmental period of deficits in language, speech, and communication.

Childhood-Onset Fluency Disorder (Stuttering): Onset during the developmental period of disturbances in normal fluency and time patterning of speech.

Social (Pragmatic) Communication Disorder: Onset during the developmental period of difficulties in the social use of verbal and nonverbal communication leading to limitations in effective communication, social participation, social relationships, academic achievement, or occupational performance.

Autism Spectrum Disorder: Deficits in social communication and social interaction. Restricted, repetitive patterns of behavior, interests, or activities.

Attention Deficit Hyperactivity Disorder: Persistence of inattention, hyperactivity-impulsivity interfering with functionality and/or development.

Specific Learning Disorder: Having difficulties learning and using academic skills.

Developmental Coordination Disorder: Coordinated motor skills below the level of the individual's chronological age and opportunity.

Tic Disorders: Recurrent episodes of sudden, rapid, recurrent, nonrhythmic motor movement or vocalization.

Schizophrenia in childhood

Defined by abnormalities in one or more of the following five domains: delusions, hallucinations, disorganized thinking (speech), grossly disorganized or abnormal motor behavior (including catatonia), and negative symptoms.

Childhood - onset schizophrenia: If disorder develops before the age 13 years.

Early-onset schizophrenia: If disorder develops before the age 18 years.

Schizophreniform disorder: Symptoms present for less than 6 months.

Schizoaffective disorder: Mood episode and symptoms of schizophrenia occur together and either preceded or are followed by at least 2 weeks of delusions or hallucinations without prominent mood symptoms.

Brief psychotic disorder:
Lasts more than 1 day and remits by 1 month.

Bipolar Disorder in children

Meet criteria for a manic episode. Manic episode may be preceded by and may be followed by hypomanic or major depressive episodes.

Bipolar II Disorder: At least 1 hypomanic episode (symptoms lasting at least 4 days) and at least 1 major depressive episode. There has never been a manic episode.

Cyclothymic Disorder: At least 1 year in children and adolescents, numerous periods of manic, hypomanic and depressive symptoms without meeting criteria for manic, hypomanic or major depressive episode.

Major Depressive Disorder: $\geq$ 5 symptoms of depression for 2-week period and at least one of the symptoms is either (1) depressed mood or (2) loss of interest or pleasure.

DMDD: Verbal/behavioral/physical aggression due to temper outburst out of the proportion to situation.

Persistent depressive Disorder: Mood is depressed or irritable for most of the day for at least 1 year for children and adolescents.

Premenstrual Dysphoric Disorder: Mood symptoms, anxiety, tension, lethargy and other symptoms present in the final week before the onset of menses, start to improve within a few days after the onset of menses, and become minimal or absent in the week postmenses.

Anxiety Disorders in children

Separation Anxiety Disorder: Inappropriate and excessive fear or anxiety concerning separation from those to whom the individual is attached.

Selective Mutism: Failure to speak in specific social situations.

Social Anxiety Disorder (Social Phobia and Specific Phobias): Specific Phobia: Fear or anxiety about a specific object or situation. Social Phobia: In children, the anxiety must occur in peer settings and not just during interactions with adults.

Panic Disorder: Recurrent unexpected panic attacks during which abrupt surge of intense fear or intense discomfort that reaches a peak within minutes from a calm state or anxious state.

Agoraphobia: Fear or anxiety of situations from which escape might seem difficult or help might not be available.

Generalized Anxiety Disorder: Excessive anxiety and worry (apprehensive expectation), for most days than not for $\geq$ 6 months, about a number of events or activities (such as work or school performance).

Obsessive Compulsive and Related Disorder

Presence of obsessions, compulsions, or both.

Body Dysmorphic Disorder: Preoccupation with ≥ 1 perceived defects or flaws in physical appearance that are not observable or appear slight to others.

Hoarding Disorder: Difficulty discarding possessions, regardless of their value. Trichotillomania: Repeated pulling out of one's hair, resulting in hair loss.

Excoriation (skin-picking) Disorders: Repeated skin picking causing skin lesions.

Trauma and Stressor Related Disorders in children

Reactive Attachment Disorder: Inhibited, emotionally withdrawn behavior toward adult caregivers.

Disinhibited Social Engagement Disorder: Child approaches and interacts with unfamiliar adults.

Posttraumatic Stress Disorder and Acute Stress Disorder: Being exposed to actual or threatened death, serious injury, or sexual violation.

Adjustment Disorders: Development of emotional or behavioral symptoms in response to an identifiable stressor or stressors.

Dissociative Disorders in children

Dissociative Identity Disorder: Two or more distinct personality states
Dissociative Amnesia:
Unable to recall important autobiographical information, usually of a traumatic or stressful event.

Depersonalization/Derealization Disorder:
Detachment or being an outside observer/Detachment with respect to surroundings.

Somatic Symptom Disorder

Preoccupation with thoughts, feelings, or behaviors associated with health concerns.

Illness Anxiety Disorder

Constantly thinking about having or acquiring a serious illness.

Conversion Disorder (Functional Neurological Symptom Disorder) in children

Symptoms are incompatible to neurological or medical conditions.
Factitious Disorder: Falsely producing signs or symptoms, injury or disease, associated with identified deception.

Feeding and Eating Disorders in children

Pica: Eating of nonnutritive, nonfood substances for at least 1 month.
Rumination Disorder: Repeated regurgitation of food over a period of at least 1 month. Regurgitated food may be re-chewed, re-swallowed, or spit out.
Avoidant/Restrictive Food Intake Disorder: An eating disorder manifested by persistent failure to meet appropriate nutritional and/or energy needs.
Anorexia Nervosa: Restriction of energy intake relative to requirements. Low weight is defined as a weight that is less than minimally normal or, for children and adolescents, less than that minimally expected.

Bulimia Nervosa: Recurrent episodes of binge eating, followed by self-induced vomiting; misuse of laxatives, diuretics, or other medications; fasting; or excessive exercise.

Binge-Eating Disorder: Recurrent episodes of binge eating, with a lack of control overeating.

Elimination Disorders in children

Enuresis: Repeated voiding of urine either involuntary or intentional.
Encopresis: Repeated passage of feces either involuntary or intentional.

Sleep-Wake Disorders in children

Insomnia: Sleep difficulty initiating and maintaining sleep.

Hypersomnolence Disorder: Excessive sleepiness despite a main sleep period lasting at least 7 hours.

Narcolepsy: Recurrent need to sleep, lapsing into sleep, or napping occurring within the same day. Occurring at least three times per week over the past 3 months.

Breathing-Related Sleep Disorders (obstructive sleep apnea hypopnea, central sleep apnea, and sleep-related hypoventilation)

Obstructive Sleep Apnea: Nocturnal breathing disturbances.

Central sleep apnea: Episodes of apneas and hypopneas.

Sleep-related hypoventilation: Episodes of decreased respiration associated with elevated CO_2 levels.

Circadian Rhythm Sleep Wake Disorders: A persistent or recurrent pattern of sleep disruption that is primarily due to an alteration of the circadian system or to a misalignment between the endogenous circadian rhythm and the sleep-wake schedule required by an individual's physical environment or social or professional schedule.

Parasomnias (NREM Sleep Arousal Disorders and Nightmare Disorder): Characterized by abnormal behavioral, experiential, or physiological events occurring in association with sleep, specific sleep stages, or sleep-wake transitions.

Non-Rapid Eye Movement Sleep Arousal Disorders: Recurrent episodes of incomplete awakening from sleep, during first third of sleep episode.

Nightmare Disorder: Repeated occurrences of remembered dreams occurring in second half of sleep that usually involve efforts to avoid threats to survival, security, or physical integrity.

Rapid Eye Movement Sleep Behavior Disorder: Repeated episodes of arousal during REM sleep, occurring > 90 minutes into sleep, which is associated with vocalization or motor behaviors.

Restless Legs Syndrome: An urge to move the legs, due to unpleasant sensations in the legs.

Gender Dysphoria

In Children (incongruence between one's experienced/expressed gender and assigned gender, of at least 6 months' duration, as manifested by at least six of the following):

Disruptive, Impulsive-Control and Conduct Disorders

Oppositional Defiant Disorder: Pattern of angry/irritable mood, argumentative/defiant behavior, or vindictiveness lasting at least 6 months as evidenced by at least four symptoms from any of the following categories and exhibited during interaction with at least one individual who is not a sibling.

Intermittent Explosive Disorder: Outbursts manifested as either: Verbal or physical aggression, occurring twice weekly, for 3 months.

Conduct Disorder: Violating basic rights of others and societal norms.

Antisocial Personality Disorder: Since the age of 15 years violating the rights of others.

Pyromania: Fire setting > 1 occasion.

Kleptomania: Recurrent impulses to steal objects not needed for personal use or for financial gain.

Substance-Related and Addictive Disorders

Continued use of substances despite cluster of cognitive, behavioral and physiological symptoms.

LIST OF SCREENING TOOLS

Mood Disorder

Survey of Wellbeing of Young Children (SWYC)/SWYC/MA: screening tool for children < 5 ½ y/o to assess developmental milestones, behavioral/emotional development, and family risk fact actors.

Available at: https://www.floatinghospital.org/The-Survey-of-Wellbeing-ofYoung-Children/Overview.aspx.

Strengths and Difficulties Questionnaire (SDQ): behavioral screening tool for youths ages 2 to 21 years. It assesses emotional symptoms, conduct problems, hyperactivity/ inattention, peer problems, and prosocial behavior.

A separate scale assesses problem presence/severity and impairment level.

Available at: www.sdqinfo.com.

Patient Health Questionnaire Modified for Teens (PHQ-9 Modified): screening tool for individuals ages 12 - 18 to assess depressive symptoms over a period of previous two weeks.

Available at: http://www.gladpc.org/

Patient Health Questionnaire (PHQ-9): screening tool for individuals ages 18 y/o and older to assess depressive symptoms over a period of previous two weeks.
Available at: http://www.phqscreeners.com/

Disruptive Mood Dysregulation Disorder (DMDD)

Disruptive Mood Dysregulation Disorder self-test:
Available at: Disruptive Mood Dysregulation Disorder: Symptom Test for Children (additudemag.com).

Substance Use

Brief Screener for Tobacco, Alcohol, and other Drugs (BSTAD) and Screening to Brief Intervention (S2BI): for adolescent patients (ages 12 - 17).
Available at: https://www.drugabuse.gov/ast/bstad/#/ and https://www.drugabuse.gov/ast/s2bi/#/
CRAFFT (Car, Relax, Alone, Forget, Friends, Trouble): a screening tool for < 21 y/o related to alcohol and drug use.
Available at: http://www.ceasar-boston.org/CRAFFT/index.php.

Anxiety

(Screen for Child Anxiety Related Disorders) – SCARED: Screening Tools|Anxiety and Depression Association of America, ADAA.
Generalized Anxiety Disorder (GAD): Screening for Generalized Anxiety Disorder (GAD)|Anxiety and Depression Association of America, ADAA.

Obsessive-Compulsive Disorder (OCD): Screening for Obsessive-Compulsive Disorder (OCD)|Anxiety and Depression Association of America, ADAA.

Panic disorder: Screening for Panic Disorder|Anxiety and Depression Association of America, ADAA.

Posttraumatic Stress Disorder (PTSD): Screening for Posttraumatic Stress Disorder (PTSD)|Anxiety and Depression Association of America, ADAA.

Social Anxiety: Screening Tools|Anxiety and Depression Association of America, ADAA.

Specific phobia: Screening for Specific Phobias|Anxiety and Depression Association of America, ADAA.

Social Phobia: Screening Tools|Anxiety and Depression Association of America, ADAA.

Autism

M-CHAT-R (Modified Checklist for Autism in Toddlers, Revised):

Schizophrenia

Child Schizophrenia Test (Self-Assessment):
Schizophrenia in Children: Is Your Child Exhibiting the Symptoms? (Test) (psycom.net).

Brief Psychiatric Rating Scale, (BPRS): Assessing Schizophrenia in Children and Adolescents (psy-ed.com).

Positive and Negative Symptom Scale, (PANSS): Assessing Schizophrenia in Children and Adolescents (psy-ed.com).

Scale for Assessment of Positive Symptoms, (SAPS), and the Scale for Assessment of Negative Symptoms, (SANS): Assessing Schizophrenia in Children and Adolescents (psy-ed.com).

Schizophrenia Test and Early Psychosis Indicator (STEPI, Version 2011.1):

Schizophrenia Test and Early Psychosis Indicator (STEPI) (counsellingresource.com).

Website from American Academy of Pediatrics (consists of list of screening and assessment tools that can be used to assess for various mental health illnesses): https://www.aap.org/en-us/advocacy-and-policy/aap-health-initiatives/Mental-Health/Documents/MH_ScreeningChart.pdf.

REFERENCES

[1] Siegel, M. (2020). Practice Parameter for the Assessment and Treatment of Psychiatric Disorders in Children and Adolescents with Intellectual Disability (Intellectual Developmental Disorder). *Journal of the American Academy of Child and Adolescent Psychiatry*, 59(4):468 - 496. https://www.jaacap.org/article/S0890-8567(19)32223-3/pdf.

[2] Volkmar, F. (2014). Practice Parameter for the Assessment and Treatment of Children and Adolescents with Autism Spectrum Disorder. *Journal of the American Academy of Child and Adolescent Psychiatry*, 53(2):237 - 257. https://www.jaacap.org/article/S0890-8567(13)00819-8/pdf.

[3] Pliszka, S. (2007). Practice Parameter for the Assessment and Treatment of Children and Adolescents with Attention-Deficit/Hyperactivity Disorder. *Journal of the American Academy of Child and Adolescent Psychiatry*, Volume 46, Issue 7, P894 - 921. https://www.jaacap.org/article/S0890-8567(09)62182-1/fulltext.

[4] Murphy, T. K. (2013). Practice Parameter for the Assessment and Treatment of Children and Adolescents with Tic Disorders. *Journal of the American Academy of Child and Adolescent Psychiatry*,

Volume 52, Issue 12, P1341 - 1359. https://www.jaacap.org/article/S0890-8567(13)00695-3/fulltext.

[5] McClellan, J. (2007). Practice Parameter for the Assessment and Treatment of Children and Adolescents with Bipolar Disorder. *Journal of the American Academy of Child and Adolescent Psychiatry*, Volume 46, Issue 1, P107 - 125. https://www.jaacap.org/article/S0890-8567(09)61968-7/fulltext.

[6] Connolly, S. D. (2007). Practice Parameter for the Assessment and Treatment of Children and Adolescents with Anxiety Disorders. *Journal of the American Academy of Child and Adolescent Psychiatry*, Volume 46, Issue 2, P267 - 283. https://www.jaacap.org/article/S0890-8567(09)61838-4/fulltext.

[7] Geller, D. A. (2012). Practice Parameter for the Assessment and Treatment of Children and Adolescents with Obsessive-Compulsive Disorder. *Journal of the American Academy of Child and Adolescent Psychiatry*, Volume 51, Issue 1, P98 - 113. https://www.jaacap.org/article/S0890-8567(11)00882-3/fulltext.

[8] Cohen, J. A. (2010). Practice Parameter for the Assessment and Treatment of Children and Adolescents with Posttraumatic Stress Disorder. *Journal of the American Academy of Child and Adolescent Psychiatry*, Volume 49, Issue 4, P414 - 430. https://www.jaacap.org/article/S0890-8567(10)00082-1/fulltext#%20.

[9] Lock, J. (2015). Practice Parameter for the Assessment and Treatment of Children and Adolescents with Eating Disorders. *Journal of the American Academy of Child and Adolescent Psychiatry*, 54(5):412 - 425. https://www.jaacap.org/article/S0890-8567(15)00070-2/pdf.

[10] Dulcan K., Mina. *Concise Guide To Child & Adolescent Psychiatry*, American Psychiatric Association, 2018.

[11] Jeste V, Dilip. *Diagnostic and Statistical Manual of Mental Disorders*, American Psychiatric Association, 2012-2013.

In: Innovations in Psychiatry
Editors: Souparno Mitra et al.
ISBN: 978-1-53619-365-7
© 2021 Nova Science Publishers, Inc.

Chapter 10

APPS FOR ATTENTION-DEFICIT HYPERACTIVITY DISORDER (ADHD)

Monika Gashi[*], *MD*

Bronx Care Health System, Department of Psychiatry,
Icahn School of Medicine, Bronx, NY, US

ABSTRACT

Attention deficit hyperactivity disorder (ADHD) is a chronic mental health condition. It can present with pattern of inattention with or without hyperactivity and or impulsivity, resulting in impairment in functioning. Some of the major functions that are affected especially in childhood are social, emotional, and cognitive development, necessary for shaping a child for adulthood. By the end this chapter you will be able to narrate the history of ADHD, its neurobiology, established treatment and available applications for patient with ADHD and their care givers, presented through a sample case.

---

[*] Corresponding Author's Email: MGashi@bronxcare.org.

INTRODUCTION

History of Attention Deficit Hyperactivity Disorder (ADHD)

Dating back to the 18th century, a Scottish physician Sir Alexander Crichton was one of the first physicians to write about the attention disorder, where "when any object of external sense, or of thought, occupies the mind in such a degree that a person does not receive a clear perception from any other one, he is said to attend to it" (Crichton, 1798). He also foresaw that the hyperactivity decreases with age, where more than 200 years later the statement continues to be correct that hyperactivity improves with age (American Psychiatric Association, 2013).

Epidemiology of ADHD

The point prevalence of ADHD in childhood is 5-8% between the ages two to seventeen, while for adult ADHD the point prevalence is 2.5% (Danielson, 2018); with an overall adult prevalence of 4.4%. Males are affected more than females, predominantly non-Hispanic and white ethnicities expressing higher prevalence than any other ethnicity or race (Kessler et al., 2006).

Neurobiology of ADHD

Attention Deficit Hyperactivity Disorder (ADHD) is a neurodevelopmental mental health condition that encompasses symptoms of hyperactivity and or inattentiveness with or without impulsivity before the age of 12 years in two different settings (American Psychiatric Association, 2013). These symptoms result in impairment of academic or occupational achievements, quality of social life as well as wellbeing of the affected individual. There are various specifiers of ADHD, including and not limited to predominantly inattentive, predominantly hyperactive, mixed, impulsive, and so forth with classification of the severity as mild, moderate or severe, depending on the interference with the quality of life of the individual.

It is postulated that areas of the brain affected resulting in symptomatology appreciated by patients with ADHD encompass: prefrontal cortex, basal ganglia and cerebellum were noted decrement in connectivity in white matter tracts continue to emerge (Curatolo et al., 2010). Furthermore, two networks that are important to revise are the default mode network and ventral network. Prefrontal cortex helps one in decision making, social behaviors, expression of self, reward anticipation and processing. Prefrontal cortex also affects cognitive behaviors such as critical thinking, memory formation and executive functioning (Siddiqui et al., 2008). While basal ganglia and cerebellum are responsible for initiation of movement and maintaining posture mediated by dopamine, which is a neurotransmitter that is released from nigro-striatal region of the basal ganglia (Krauel et al., 2010). The default mode network involves lateral parietal cortex which is preoccupied with internal cues, hence active at rest (Hale et al., 2014). Therefore affected individuals with ADHD are unable to delay gratification, thus unable to wait for bigger prizes and a need immediate relish. Due to decrease in visual-spatial attention and goal-oriented tasks, affected individual with ADHD is more prone to accidents, such as tripping in flat surfaces, head injuries, thus inept and known as being "clumsy." While the day dreaming involves the default mode network making it hard to be attentive to other stimuli. The ventral network involves inferior frontal gyrus, anterior insula and temporoparietal junction, makes it hard for the affected individual to shift attention from one task to another unexpected but relevant stimuli (McCarthy et al. 2013). For instance while a child or adult is playing videogames, and their parent or partner asks them to do something else; they may not notice them; thus can result in being perceived as "ignorant;" "dismissive;" "defiant;" when in reality the individual did not notice the other person standing or talking to them, ergo resulting in miscommunication and conflicts in their relationship.

Comorbidities

ADHD is highly comorbid with other psychiatric conditions. Up to two-thirds of patients with ADHD will meet criteria for another psychiatric condition; 50% of patients will have oppositional defiant disorder, 15% to 20% will have a mood disorder such as major depressive disorder or bipolar disorder, and 20% to 25% will have an anxiety disorder such as generalized anxiety disorder. Psychotic disorders such as schizophrenia can be present but are less common when compared to other choices (Biender et al., 1991).

SAMPLE CASE

Johnny is a 9-year-old male with history of inattention, running frequently into things, and hurting self, at times he trips on the floor, despite no toys being around. He frequently needs redirection by his parents, and teacher frequently call his parents to school due to his inability to sit, talking out of turn, disrupting the class, easily irritable, and slow to follow redirection. What is the most likely diagnosis?

After obtaining Vanderbilt scale for teachers and parents as well as Conner's parenting scale and Conner's Teachers scale, which are scales that rate one's functionality at home and at school, in two different settings. It was concluded that Johnny's most likely diagnosis is Attention Deficit Hyperactivity disorder, predominantly hyperactive, moderate.

Johnny's parents do wonder if ADHD is linked with any other conditions?

The physician further informs Johnny's parents that untreated ADHD results in academic underachievement, despite the normal intelligence, as well as has increased risk of anxiety, mood dysregulation, resulting in increased risk of substance use such as marijuana, alcohol, nicotine and other substances (Merikangas et al., 2010).

Johnny's parents ask the provider about the chance of ADHD continuing into adulthood?

The physician psycho-educates the parents regarding the prevalence of ADHD in children being less than 9%, while in adults about 4% (Merikangas et al., 2010; NCS, 2005).

Johnny's parents wanted to understand better how does this "ADHD" related to his clumsiness?

The physician kindly started describing the interconnection of different parts of the brain being affected which help with his organization, his daily activities, his functioning in school being able to remain attentive and absorb the information provided to him by teachers and his ability to achieve his full potential.

After synthesizing all the education regarding ADHD, Johnny's parents were wondering about the modalities of treatment of ADHD?

Moreover, the physician reports that there are FDA approved medications: on label and off label medications such as stimulant (amphetamine salts and methylphenidate); non-stimulant medications (SSRI (atomoxetine); NDRI (buproprione)- off label; alpha agonists (clonidine, guanfacine- off label)) as well as parental interventions and individual psychotherapy to provide structure for the affected individual.

TREATMENT OF ADHD

Doctor Charles Bradly was the first physician from Rhode Island in 1937 who coined the response of treatment with stimulants for ADHD in children (Bradly, 1937). There are various treatments that are currently available, pharmacologic and non-pharmacological, FDA approved and off label use. There are different classes of medications, such as stimulants and non-stimulant medications, as well as cognitive behavioral therapy that require structure both at home and at school. There have been various studies conducted to investigate the best treatment approaches regarding ADHD with medication alone, or medication and structure, parenting education versus structure therapy alone for 6-8 years. In the end it was noted that the highest dropout rate of patient population with ADHD came from: single parent house hold, lower education and lower socio-economic status, resulting in higher academic impact, substance use disorder and homelessness (Molina et al., 2009).

Table 1. Medications for ADHD

Medications Approved by the FDA for ADHD (Alphabetical by Class)

Generic Class/Brand Name	Dose Form	Typical Starting Dose	FDA Max/Day	Off-Label Max/Day	Comments
Amphetamine preparations					
Short-acting					
Adderall*	5, 7.5, 10, 12.5, 15, 20, 30 mg tab	3–5 y: 2.5 mg q.d.; ≥6 y: 5 mg q.d.–b.i.d.	40 mg	>50 kg: 60 mg	Short-acting stimulants often used as initial treatment in small children (<16 kg), but have disadvantage of b.i.d.–t.i.d. dosing to control symptoms throughout day
Dexedrine*	5 mg cap	3–5 y: 2.5 mg q.d.			
DextroStat*	5, 10 mg cap	≥6 y: 5 mg q.d.–b.i.d.			
Long-acting					
Dexedrine Spansule	5, 10, 15 mg cap	≥6 y: 5–10 mg q.d.–b.i.d.	40 mg	>50 kg: 60 mg	Longer acting stimulants offer greater convenience, confidentiality, and compliance with single daily dosing but may have greater problematic effects on evening appetite and sleep Adderall XR cap may be opened and sprinkled on soft foods
Adderall XR	5, 10, 15, 20, 25, 30 mg cap	≥6 y: 10 mg q.d.	30 mg	>50 kg: 60 mg	
Lisdexamfetamine	30, 50, 70 mg cap	30 mg q.d.	70 mg	Not yet known	
Methylphenidate preparations					
Short-acting					
Focalin	2.5, 5, 10 mg cap	2.5 mg b.i.d.	20 mg	50 mg	Short-acting stimulants often used as initial treatment in small children (<16 kg) but have disadvantage of b.i.d.–t.i.d. dosing to control symptoms throughout day
Methylin*	5, 10, 20 mg tab	5 mg b.i.d.	60 mg	>50 kg: 100 mg	
Ritalin*	5, 10, 20 mg	5 mg b.i.d.	60 mg	>50 kg: 100 mg	
Intermediate-acting					
Metadate ER	10, 20 mg cap	10 mg q.a.m.	60 mg	>50 kg: 100 mg	Longer acting stimulants offer greater convenience, confidentiality, and compliance with single daily dosing but may have greater problematic effects on evening appetite and sleep Metadate CD and Ritalin LA caps may be opened and sprinkled on soft food
Methylin ER	10, 20 mg cap	10 mg q.a.m.	60 mg	>50 kg: 100 mg	
Ritalin SR*	20 mg	10 mg q.a.m.	60 mg	>50 kg: 100 mg	
Metadate CD	10, 20, 30, 40, 50, 60 mg	20 mg q.a.m.	60 mg	>50 kg: 100 mg	
Ritalin LA	10, 20, 30, 40 mg	20 mg q.a.m.	60 mg	>50 kg: 100 mg	
Long-acting					
Concerta	18, 27, 36, 54 mg cap	18 mg q.a.m.	72 mg	108 mg	Swallow whole with liquids Nonabsorbable tablet shell may be seen in stool.
Daytrana patch	10, 15, 20, 30 mg patches	Begin with 10 mg patch q.d., then titrate up by patch strength	30 mg	Not yet known	
Focalin XR	5, 10, 15, 20 mg cap	5 mg q.a.m.	30 mg	50 mg	
Selective norepinephrine reuptake inhibitor					
Atomoxetine					Not a schedule II medication
Strattera	10, 18, 25, 40, 60, 80, 100 mg cap	Children and adolescents <70 kg: 0.5 mg/kg/day for 4 days; then 1 mg/kg/day for 4 days; then 1.2 mg/kg/day	Lesser of 1.4 mg/kg or 100 mg	Lesser of 1.8 mg/kg or 100 mg	Consider if active substance abuse or severe side effects of stimulants (mood lability, tics); give q.a.m. or divided doses b.i.d. (effects on late evening behavior); do not open capsule; monitor closely for suicidal thinking and behavior, clinical worsening, or unusual changes in behavior

Note: FDA = U.S. Food and Drug Administration; ADHD = attention-deficit/hyperactivity disorder.
* Generic formulation available.

APPS FOR ADHD

Millennial age group are known for utilizing technology whether in school setting, socially with one another or at work. One of the means that many application developers have attempted to innovate are to meet their clientele's expectations, that is reach out to them though media via different applications. Patients with attention deficit hyperactivity disorder are notorious to be forgetful, easily distractible, affecting their academic performance and other life time achievements if not addressed timely. While, when it comes to playing video-games they are excellent, due to various stimuli and frequent reward systems within the games.

In order to help the patients and their families with their daily activities, ensuring parents, teachers and student engagement, though no evidence base yet nor FDA approval, below are some applications that have platforms of use by more than 9 million teachers; students; parents, nationally and internationally in more than 30 countries for some of the applications. Below you will find the names of the applications, their use, with fees, and availability for various devices.

Table 2. Apps for ADHD

Application	What is it used for?	Evidence Based	FDA approved	Fee/Availability
"Class Dojo"	Collaboration between teachers and parents on refining behavior; class participation and specific positive feedback from teachers. Parents can opt in to obtain further info on child's behavior in real time.	Not yet.	Not yet.	Free/iOS, Android
"Here Comes the Bus"	Helps parents to track the bus their child takes; as well as ensure the child got off on the right stop.	Not yet.	Not yet.	Free/iOS, Android
"Study Stack"	Helps create fun ways for the child to learn and recall information through a gaming process.	Not yet.	Not yet.	Free/iOS, Android
"dexteria"	Help refine the fine motor skills from kindergarten to adulthood.	Not yet	Not yet	$3.99/iOS, Android

Table 2. (Continued)

Application	What is it used for?	Evidence Based	FDA approved	Fee/Availability
"Kahoot"	Teachers input their questions and answers while students utilize web browsers as "buzzer" to engage along with other peers like a trivia game.	Not yet	Not yet	Free/iOS, Android
"photomath"	Helps children with ADHD tutoring them and guiding the children and adolescents under supervision step by step to the final solution	Not yet	Not yet	Basic version: Free/iOS, Android Supporter version: $ 0.99 per month/iOS, Android
"grade Proof"	Checks spelling, grammar, and formatting errors, when children with ADHD are writing assignments, as dyslexia and dysgraphia are common conditions that co-occur.	Not yet	Not yet	Basic version: Free/iOS, Premium: $ 9.99 per month/iOS
"WHAAM app"	Improves collaboration between family, provider and teachers regarding Applied behavioral application; planned interventions and collecting behavioral data reported	Not yet	Not yet	Unknown.

CONCLUSION

Access to technology, such as mobile devices, ipads, laptops, and internet have resulted in vicissitudes in the social functioning and societal expectations. The hunt for newer and more personalized modalities to engage parents and their children in daily activities, monitor symptoms and further advice pursuit continues. The newest trend regarding ADHD applications involves many platforms available for both the caregivers and the affected individual, but thus far nothing has been evidence-based nor FDA approved.

REFERENCES

American Psychiatric Association. (2013). *Diagnostic and statistical manual of mental disorders* (5th ed.). Arlington, VA: Author.

Biederman, J., Newcorn J., Sprich S. Comorbidity of attention deficit hyperactivity disorder with conduct, depressive, anxiety, and other disorders. *Am J Psychiatry* 148:564-577, 1991.

Bradley, C. (1937) The behavior of children receiving benzedrine. *Am J Psychiatry* 94:577-585.

Crichton, A. (1798) An inquiry into the nature and origin of mental derangement: comprehending a concise system of the physiology and pathology of the human mind and a history of the passions and their effects. Cadell T. Jr, Davies W., London [Reprint: Crichton A. (2008) An inquiry into the nature and origin of mental derangement. On attention and its diseases. *J Atten Disord* 12:200-204].

Curatolo, P., D'Agati, E., and Moavero, R. (2010). The neurobiological basis of ADHD. *Italian journal of pediatrics,* 36(1), 79. https://doi.org/10.1186/1824-7288-36-79.

Danielson, M. L., Bitsko, R. H., Ghandour, R. M., Holbrook, J. R., Kogan, M. D., and Blumberg, S. J. (2018). Prevalence of Parent-Reported ADHD Diagnosis and Associated Treatment Among U.S. Children and Adolescents, 2016. *Journal of clinical child and adolescent psychology: the official journal for the Society of Clinical Child and Adolescent Psychology,* American Psychological Association, Division 53, 47(2), 199-212. https://doi.org/10.1080/15374416.2017.1417860.

Hale, T. S., Kane, A. M., Kaminsky, O., Tung, K. L., Wiley, J. F., McGough, J. J., Kaplan, J. T. (2014). Visual network asymmetry and default mode network function in ADHD: An fmri study. Frontiers in Psychiatry, 5. doi: https://doi.org/10.3389/fpsyt.2014.00081

Kessler, R. C., Adler L., Barkley R., Biederman J., Conners C. K., Demler O., Faraone S. V., Greenhill L. L., Howes M. J., Secnik K., Spencer T., Ustun T. B., Walters E. E., Zaslavsky A. M. The prevalence and correlates of adult ADHD in the United States: results from the

National Comorbidity Survey Replication. *Am J Psychiatry.* 2006 Apr; 163(4):716-23. PMID: 16585449.

Krauel, K., Feldhaus H. C., Simon A., Rehe C., Glaser M., Flechtner H. H., et al., Increased echogenicity of the substantia nigra in children and adolescents with attention-deficit/hyperactivity disorder. *Biol Psychiatry.* 2010; 68:352-8. doi: https://10.1016/j.biopsych.2010.01.013.

Lange, K. W., Reichl, S., Lange, K. M., Tucha, L., and Tucha, O. (2010). The history of attention deficit hyperactivity disorder. *Attention deficit and hyperactivity disorders*, 2(4), 241-255. https://doi.org/10.1007/s12402-010-0045-8.

McCarthy, H., Skokauskas, N., Mulligan, A., Donohoe, G., Mullins, D., Kelly, J., Frodl, T. (2013). Attention network Hypoconnectivity with default and AFFECTIVE Network HYPERCONNECTIVITY in adults diagnosed With attention-deficit/hyperactivity disorder in childhood. *JAMAPsychiatry*, 70(12), 1329. doi: 10.1001/jamapsychiatry.2013.2174

Merikangas, K. R., He J. P., Burstein M., Swanson S. A., Avenevoli S., Cui L., Benjet C., Georgiades K., Swendsen J. Lifetime prevalence of mental disorders in U.S. adolescents: results from the National Comorbidity Survey Replication-Adolescent Supplement (NCS-A). *J Am Acad Child Adolesc Psychiatry.* 2010 Oct; 49(10):980-9. PMID: 20855043.

Merlo, G., Chiazzese G., Sanches-Ferreira M., Chifari A., Seta L., McGee C., Mirisola A., Giammusso I. The WHAAM application: a tool to support the evidence-based practice in the functional behaviour assessment. *J Innov Health Inform.* 2018; 25(2):63-70. https://www.additudemag.com/slideshows/adhd-back-to-school-apps/.

Molina, B., Hinshaw, S. P., Swanson, J. M., Arnold, L. E., Vitiello, B., Jensen, P. S., Epstein, J. N., Hoza, B., Hechtman, L., Abikoff, H. B., Elliott, G. R., Greenhill, L. L., Newcorn, J. H., Wells, K. C., Wigal, T., Gibbons, R. D., Hur, K., Houck, P. R., and MTA Cooperative Group (2009). The MTA at 8 years: prospective follow-up of children treated for combined-type ADHD in a multisite study. *Journal of the*

American Academy of Child and Adolescent Psychiatry, 48(5), 484-500. https://doi.org/10.1097/CHI.0b013e31819c23d0.

NCS-A Lifetime and 12M prevalence estimates. 2005; https://www.hcp.med.harvard.edu/ncs/.

Pliszka, S., The AACAP Work Group on Quality Issues. Practice Parameter for the Assessment and Treatment of Children and Adolescents with Attention-Deficit/Hyperactivity Disorder. *AACAP Official Action*, Volume 46, ISSUE 7, P894-921, July 01, 2007. doi: https://doi.org/10.1097/chi.0b013e318054e724.

Siddiqui, S. V., Chatterjee, U., Kumar, D., Siddiqui, A., & Goyal, N. (2008). Neuropsychology of prefrontal cortex. *Indian journal of psychiatry*, 50(3), 202-208. https://doi.org/10.4103/0019-5545.43634.

In: Innovations in Psychiatry
Editors: Souparno Mitra et al.

ISBN: 978-1-53619-365-7
© 2021 Nova Science Publishers, Inc.

Chapter 11

APPS FOR SUBSTANCE USE DISORDERS

Kiran Jose[*], *MD*

*BronxCare Health System, Department of Psychiatry,
Icahn School of Medicine, Bronx, NY, US*

ABSTRACT

In this chapter, we discuss the role of mobile health apps that facilitate recovery from substance use disorders.

We start the chapter by understanding the definition and the diagnostic criteria used for substance use disorders along with some recent epidemiological data. We then discuss how mobile apps incorporates pharmacological and behavioral interventions to help patients with substance use disorders.

Benefits and shortcomings of these mobile phone-based health inventions are acknowledged as well and further studies are required to gauge the efficacy and functionality of these apps.

---

[*] Corresponding Author's E-mail: KJose@bronxcare.org.

Addiction and Use of Applications

Addiction is a medical disorder, a complex condition that affects the brain and is manifested by compulsive substance use despite harmful consequence.

Individuals with severe substance use disorder tend to have an increased focus on using specific substances such as alcohol or drugs, to the point that it takes over their life. Generally, addiction develops over the following states: occasional use, recreational use, regular use and eventually, addiction. Individuals with substance use disorder are noted to have distorted thinking, behavior, and body functions. Studies report changes in the brain's wiring results in causing intense cravings and the inability to stop the drug use. There are several biological and environmental risk factors identified, along with the search for genetic variations that contribute to the development and progression of the disorder.

This knowledge is useful especially for the development of prevention and treatment approaches that reduce the impact of drug use on individuals, families, and communities.

According to the 2019 National Survey on Drug Use and Health, among people age 12 years and older, 60. 1 percent used a substance (tobacco, alcohol, illicit drugs). Among 20.4 million people aged 12 or older with past year Substance use disorder in 2019, 71.7 percent had a past year alcohol use disorder, 40.7 percent had a past year illicit drug use disorder, and 11.8 percent had both an alcohol use disorder and an illicit drug use disorder in the past year. Although addiction is a chronic relapsing condition, it can be successfully managed with medication treatment along with behavioral therapies. As per the 2019 National Survey on Drug Use and Health, 2.1 million substance users received treatment at a self-help group, 1.7 million received treatment at a rehabilitation facility as an outpatient, 1.3 million received treatment at a mental health center as an outpatient, and 1.0 million received treatment as a rehabilitation facility as an inpatient, and 948,000 received treatment a private doctor's office.

SAMPLE CASE

Mr. C is a 25-year-old Hispanic male with past psychiatric history of anxiety, depression, and polysubstance use disorder. He is domiciled in his uncle's apartment, works as a part time construction worker and is a father to his 2-year-old daughter. He has been living with his uncle for the past 4 years and maintains good relationship with his daughter's mother who lives separately.

He grew up in Puerto Rico till the age of 10 and migrated to United States with his parents. He was first introduced to Marijuana and alcohol at the age of 14 in high school. He started using marijuana on a regular basis for the next two years which started affecting his school and personal life. What started as an occasional, recreational use became part of his everyday life and he was further introduced to cocaine, heroin and benzodiazepines towards the end of high school. Although he was able to complete high school, he was unable to further his education due to the financial situation at home and his polysubstance use.

It was at this point that Mr. C's dad committed suicide, which played a crucial role in his life. He started drinking alcohol more frequently along with his existing substance use. He was unable to cope with his father's death and he resorted to drugs as a way to escape from reality. After more than 1 year of continuous substance use, he was able to start working at an auto mechanic shop at the age of 21 but was unable to keep his job due to his inability to concentrate, increased craving and low functionality at work. He had difficulty prioritizing tasks at work and was in constant need to be intoxicated to alleviate his anxiety and depression. He started having difficulty financially supporting himself and was unable to care for his daughter. On the behest of his family, he voluntarily admitted himself to inpatient detox and rehabilitation program, which he quit after 13 days due to some 'personal reasons'.

After this admission, he had 2 other inpatient admissions which he was unable to finish successfully. After several relapses, he overdosed on heroin, at which point, he was admitted to inpatient psychiatric facility and was further transferred to a detox program. His family was involved during this visit, he was more motivated at this admission and has been successfully attending groups and individual therapy on a regular basis. He also started treatment for his depression and anxiety and has been compliant with his medications. He in being set up with outpatient psychiatric clinic affiliated with the Hospital.

ESTABLISHED TREATMENT FOR ADDICTION

1. Medication assisted treatment
   Pharmacological intervention for addiction is dependent on the substance used by the individual. Commonly used medications include, Naltrexone, Vivitrol, Acamprosate, Naloxone, methadone and Buprenorphine.
2. Motivational interviewing
   A collaborative, autonomy-supporting approach where clinicians help patients explore and resolve their ambivalence about changing behaviors that are not healthy. Several techniques are used to build rapport and provide support to the patient in a non-judgmental manner.
3. Cognitive behavioral therapy
   Helps patients understand their biased cognitions and factors related to substance use. The primary goal includes helping them acquire the ability to understand their risk factors for substance use, and develop effective coping responses to their urges.
4. Addiction counselling
   This is a commonly used treatment for substance use disorder that is formatted for both the individual and group setting. The counselling sessions focus primarily on learning strategies to avoid urges, situations and trigger factors that lead to substance use. It also incorporates several principles of 12-step programs like Alcoholic anonymous and several psychotherapies such as

supportive, behavioral, insight-oriented and cognitive behavioral therapy.
5. Twelve step facilitation
This is the most popular intervention which has shown success in alcohol use. It is an intervention provided by a clinician that introduces patients to the 12-step philosophy in an individual patient format. This is delivered over 12 sessions, which begin by encouraging participation, followed by steps that include reviewing and recover-oriented activity planning.

MARS (MOBILE APPS RATING SCALE)

The use of smartphone has grown exponentially in the recent years. Concurrently, increasing number of individuals use smartphone apps related to health and well-being. The MARS is an objective and reliable tool that was developed to assess and categorize the quality of mobile health apps. Since its development, the rating scale has been used as a checklist for the development of new high-quality health apps. This rating tool measures five broad categories of criteria that includes engagement, functionality, aesthetics, information quality, as well as the app subjective quality.

APPS FOR ADDICTION

Despite advances in scientific research, we do not have a comprehensive understanding of why some people develop addiction to drugs or how it alters the brain to foster compulsive drug use. According to current research, several biological and environmental factors play a pivotal role in development and progression of addiction overall. Based on this knowledge, effective prevention and treatment approaches have been successful in reducing the toll that drug use takes on individuals, families, and communities. Factors such as cost of care, lack of insurance coverage, fear of losing a job and stigma surrounding addiction are some reasons that prevent people from seeking care with existing evidence-based interventions.

In the last several years, mobile phone-based health inventions have been on the rise. This has been shown to have potential promise to optimize the delivery of care for persons with substance use with minimal disruption to an individual's regular schedule and to health systems. In an effort to increase access to recovery resources, evidence-based research has been intertwined with technology to provide treatment and recovery resources for addiction. Here, individuals have frequent access to support and connection with the mind, body and spirit. These apps provide venues where one can track personal sobriety, virtual journal, monitor triggers and connect with peers who are going through the same journey.

Cell phone apps created to target alcohol, benzodiazepine, cocaine, crack/cocaine, crystal methamphetamine and heroin use are analyzed and compared based on the mobile apps rating scale (MARS) and content analysis. A systematic search of iTunes and Google Play app stores for free low-cost apps facilitating recovery was conducted, where the results were evaluated based on functionality, aesthetics and quality of the information provided for their users. Mobile phone-based health interventions provide a unique, flexible, and affordable approach to improving health outcomes. Some effective ways of reducing the burden of substance use disorders using technology includes smartphone aps, short message services (SMS) text messaging, and interactive voice response. Smartphone apps promise to enhance the reach of evidence-based interventions such as cognitive behavior therapy, contingency management, and therapeutic education system for individuals with substance use disorders while ensuring minimal disruption to the health system. Due to existing barriers such as cost, stigma and lack of health care provider availability, smartphone apps have been gaining popularity among individuals with substance use disorders to reduce alcohol and illicit substance use.

Due to increasing popularity of smartphone apps that facilitate recovery from alcohol and illicit substances, a systematic search was conducted in 2018 that included information from apps on iTune App Store, Google Play, PubMed, Google Scholar, and PsychInfo.

The MARS rating scale was successfully incorporated to assess the quality of the smartphone apps. The classification domain is a descriptive survey of app price, platform, rating and technical features such as password protection and log-in protocols. Out of the 74 apps that met the inclusion criteria, majority of the apps were targeted towards alcohol use (n = 40), 6 were for opioid use and none focused on cocaine, crack/cocaine or methamphetamine use. Apps that had the highest average MARS score included SoberWorx (4.20), Recovery Today Magazine (3.77), Sober Grid (3.75), and Addicaid: Addiction Recovery and Support (3.64). The lowest-ranking apps included Sick Not Stupid (1.64), Sober Day Recovery App (1.71), and Stop Drinking Alcohol Now (1.75).

The highly rated apps were further analyzed to understanding the features that attributed to increased engagement and clinical impact among users. Features that contributed to efficacy of these apps included their innovative design, content in initial assessments, tracking substance use and its consequences, access to peer support as per geospatial positioning and allowing individuals with substance use disorders and their family members to locate 12-step group meetings, treatment programs and other services. The two apps that utilized evidence-based approach initial assessment were The Saying When and Alcohol Tracker apps. The Saying When app included an initial baseline assessment of individual's drinking patterns, tracking their use, setting goals and providing information regarding community resources. The Alcohol Tracker app utilized the Alcohol Use Disorders Identification Test and Functional Analysis of Addictive Behaviors to notify users regarding their alcohol consumption based National Institute of Health and Care Excellence UK Guidelines. The app that was most focused on facilitation of peer support was Sober Grid which allowed users to share posts on their experiences and insights with regards to recovery. This app also connected users to their peers online and in-person, and also allowed clinicians and health systems to provide online support. The highest rated app was SoberWox, which provided peer support, connected users to treatment centers, addiction counseling and sober living homes. This app also allowed family members to locate additional resources within the area.

Out of the few government-initiated apps that offered risk reduction measures for individuals with substance use disorders was STOP OD NYC. The app provided information about opioids and instructions on administering naloxone. It also provided users information regarding risk-reduction and linked users with pharmacies, harm reduction programs and centers providing free of cost naloxone. One of the promising apps called FlexDek MAT that was designed for SAMHSA was targeted towards opioid treatment but had limited resources and lacked basic functionality.

Despite an increase in number of apps available for substance use disorders, no evidence of incorporating evidence-based approach was found. These apps also lacked functionality where most of the peer support forums were unresponsive. Although several apps promised linking users to treatment programs and providers, the information provided were not updated and were not tailored to uninsured or Medicaid-insured users.

CBT (Cognitive Behavioral Therapy) and relapse prevention strategies are also found to be an essential and effective part of treatment of substance use disorders. However, majority of the apps did not utilize this in the services being provided. The apps analyzed in this study were assessed for integration of evidence-based psychotherapeutic and pharmacological approach to substance use disorder. Based on current analysis, further studies are necessary to measure the effectiveness of using cell phone apps for substance use disorders. More evidence-based approach along with improved access to harm-reduction resources, treatment programs and connecting users to primary care-based treatment would enhance the use of cell phone apps in substance use disorder.

REFERENCES

[1] NIDA. 2020, July 20. *Preface.* Retrieved from https://www.drugabuse.gov/publications/drugs-brains-behavior-science-addiction/preface on 2020, November 10.

[2] Use, K. S. (2019). Mental Health Indicators in the United States: *Results from the 2018 National Survey on Drug Use and Health.* HHS Pub No. PEP19 5068, NSDUH Series H-54. Rockville, MD. Center for Behavioral Health Statistics and Quality, Substance Abuse and Mental Health Services Administration.

[3] Liu, J. F. and Li, J. X. (2018). Drug addiction: a curable mental disorder? *Acta pharmacologica Sinica,* 39(12), 1823 - 1829. https://doi.org/10.1038/s41401-018-0180-x.

[4] Barry, C. L., McGinty, E. E., Pescosolido, B. A. and Goldman, H. H. (2014). Stigma, discrimination, treatment effectiveness, and policy: public views about drug addiction and mental illness. *Psychiatric services,* (Washington, DC), 65(10), 1269 - 1272. https://doi.org/10.1176/appi.ps.201400140.

[5] Tofighi, B., Chemi, C., Ruiz-Valcarcel, J., Hein, P. and Hu, L. (2019). Smartphone Apps Targeting Alcohol and Illicit Substance Use: Systematic Search in in Commercial App Stores and Critical Content Analysis. *JMIR mHealth and uHealth,* 7(4), e11831. https://doi.org/10.2196/11831.

In: Innovations in Psychiatry ISBN: 978-1-53619-365-7
Editors: Souparno Mitra et al. © 2021 Nova Science Publishers, Inc.

Chapter 12

PSYCHOLOGICAL TESTING TOOLS

Khai Tran[*], MD
BronxCare Health System, Department of Psychiatry
Icahn School of Medicine
Bronx, NY, US

ABSTRACT

With the advancement of technology, as of 2020, the smart phone penetration rate globally is 45.4%. The accessibility of the information highway made it easier to communicate between patient and provider but also allows ease of access to educational information. In this chapter, we look at the smart phone applications that would allow screening and evaluation for mental disorder as well as the near future direction that would streamline care for patient and provider.

---

[*] Corresponding Author's Email: ktran@bronxcare.org.

THE HISTORY OF PSYCHIATRIC ASSESSMENT AND DIAGNOSIS

Modern psychiatry has deep rooted history with Sigmund Freud and psychoanalysis. However, at the time of Freud, the focus was to recognize the symptoms and understand the manifestation of the hidden unconscious rather than treating a diagnosis. The dictum of no treatment without diagnosis demanded classification categories for recognizing mental illnesses. Philippe Pinel and August Heinroth set forth initial scientific sets of symptoms to classify a disease. It wasn't until 1883 when Emil Kraepelin created his version of disease classification that became the standard at the time. Some of his works remained until today in the current DSM version. He was widely recognized for setting the diagnostic differentiation between psychotic and mood disorder. In 1945, Willing Menninger published the Technical Medical Bulletin #203 which served as the predecessor to the first DSM version. His work was a combination of Freud's and Kraepelin's work to set new diagnostic categories for manic-depressive disorder and psychotic disorder. In 1952, George Raines and the American Psychiatric Association put forth the first edition of the Diagnostic and Statistical Manual of Mental Disorders, commonly known as the DSM series. The DSM-I was built closely to the Medical Bulletin 203 with more comprehensive diagnostic criteria. The DSM series underwent numerous revisions throughout the year to its newest edition the DSM-5 which serves as the current diagnostic standard in psychiatry.

With the indicative criteria set forth by the DSM series as the gold standard for diagnosing a specific mental illness, several assessment tools became available for mental health workers to utilize. There are currently over 75 different psychiatric assessment tools and rating scales to be used in both adult and child/adolescent population to address every mental disorder listed in the DSM. These assessments can be separated in 7 different categories:

1. General psychiatric health: for routine monitoring during health checkups, there are Kessler series, Patient Stress Questionnaire, M3 Check list
2. Depression: Patient Health Questionnaire is frequently for symptoms of depression. SIG E CAPS, a mnemonic created by Carey Gross from Massachusetts General Hospital is commonly used to assess depression
3. Bipolar disorder: STABLE Resources, Mood disorder Questionnaire, Bipolar Spectrum Diagnostic Scale are used, similarly the mnemonic DIGFAST is also utilized
4. Anxiety Disorder: for screening of generalized anxiety, OCD, panic disorder, PTSD, there are many tools such as GAD-7, PCL-5, HAM-A, YBOCS
5. Trauma: Life event Checklist can help identify major sources of trauma or distress that would result in PTSD or specific anxiety disorder
6. Suicide Risk: SAFE-T, C-SSRS, ASQ, Stanley-Brown are used to screen for risk of suicide or assist in suicide prevention
7. Drug and substance use: Alcohol use Disorder Identification Test, National Institute on Drug Abuse NIDAMED, CAGE, AUDIT-C, DAST-10, CIWA-AR, CIWA-b, COWS are all used to screen for substance use, withdrawal symptoms

THE EXPLOSION OF MOBILE TECHNOLOGY AND THE TRANSITION OF MENTAL HEALTH MONITORING

Within the last 2 decades, the advancement in mobile technologies have bloomed significantly with more than 5.2 billion people who have access to smart phones and the internet. They have unlimited access to resources, people and services in the palm of their hands. With it, the digital mobile application technology has also one of the most demanded markets. In terms of medical care, available mobile health applications are ranging from self-help to daily assessment to telecommunication with primary health care provider. With the accessibility of this information, it made clinicians wonder how interested their patients were in this data. A survey was conducted in Massachusetts General Hospital which demonstrated that more than 60% of their patients were "very" or "extremely" interested in utilizing mobile devices as a means to receive updates, education and communication with their care providers and more than 60% of people who own smart phones have downloaded and used one of the health apps. Currently there are hundreds of thousands of health related apps available on both the Play Store and the App Store. Despite the availability and the rapid rate of utilization, these apps' efficacy, reliability remained questionable due to the fact that many of these apps that are designed for the purpose of diagnosis and treatment were designed without the involvement of a professional health care worker or have reliable utilization of current research. Another pit fall of having availability of information is that the level of education of the user may not be adequate to have proper understanding and appropriate utilization of the information provided.

The current model for diagnosing mental disorders relies heavily on the recognition of signs and symptoms of a specific disorder; however, this does not incorporate the relevant neurobiological, socioeconomic aspects into the illness. This system is an impediment to the advancement of psychiatry as well. Assessment, diagnosis, formulation, treatment and follow-ups are critical in mental health care and regular communication is instrumental to the outcome of effective care treatment. Unlike medical illness, psychiatric disorders are not diagnosed based on physical exams, lab tests or diagnostic imaging to establish a diagnosis; instead, they rely heavily on mental status exam, psychiatrists' observation and clinical judgment, patient's cooperation and self-reports. Even with years of training, evolution of diagnostic guide lines, refined assessment tools, the formulation remained subjective depending on the psychiatrist. Furthermore, presenting symptoms are based solely on the patient's recollection and perceptions and their ability to recall information during clinical interviews leading to inaccurate reporting and biases.

Currently there are over 50,000 mobile apps that relate to mental health. These apps can be divided into 3 categories: physician centered, patient centered, and physician – patient intercommunication.

1. Physician centered apps: at the current time, mental health apps and are mostly direct translation from their pen-paper counter parts. MedCalc allows user to input data for assessment tools such as CIWA-AR, CIWA-b, COWS, 4 A's for delirium etc., anything that requires simple data input for a summation of scores and provide recommendation based on score. Epocrates, Medscape are basic searchable data bases for information gathering. Some of these apps are preset algorithms that would provide differential diagnoses that are closely related to the "subjective self reported" symptoms, some even provide with potential treatment option with psychopharmacology. These may be more helpful to providers that are less experienced such as in primary care rather than psychiatrists.
2. Patient centered apps: there are tens of thousands apps available for regular consumers to download and use, some are free and some requires one time payment. Most are unsupported by any professional health care provider.

    Many researches were conducted to examine the efficacy of these applications. One research conducted by Marshall etc al in 2019 looked at specifically the apps that were available to address anxiety and depression with therapeutic treatment. They looked at 293 apps that fit their inclusion criteria and found that only 3.14% had research that supported their claim of effectiveness, 30% have "expert development" input, and 20% were associated with a government, academic institution or medical facility. This demonstrated the need for much more research, collaboration and testing prior to being available for usage. Despite poor results, some of the apps were able to demonstrate good potential and free to use such as WellWave, PeerFIT, FOCUS, Mindsurf, PTSD Coach, MoodMission.

3. Physician – Patient communication: at this time, communication between patient and health care provider are basic secure messaging apps such as Doximity, TigerConnect. This is an underdeveloped area that has vast potential to elevate mental health care to the next level through health promoting education such as medication compliance, diet, exercises; intervention and prevention exercises as well as reduction of numbers of face to face sessions. Comprehensive feed backs would also allow care providers to have thorough understanding of patient's daily lives objectively to formulate a better treatment plan.

Table 1. Samples of general mental health apps and their specific designs

Applications name	Purpose
MedCalc, MDCalc	User input point of care apps for medical equations, algorithms and guideline
Epocrates, UpToDate, VisualDx	Medical database for medical database and up to date treatments guidelines and diagnoses
Doximity, Tiger Connect, Figure 1	Secure communication apps
MY3, notOK	Suicide prevention via self design safety plans
What'sup, MoodKit	Mood improvement based on CBT
Quit That!, Twenty-four hours a day	Addiction habit, triggering behaviors tracking apps for addiction
Mindshift, Self help for anxiety management	Coping strategies, emotional diary for anxiety
iMood, eMoods	Mood tracking apps designed for bipolar disorders
Talkspace, Happify, Moodtools	Coping supports, therapy recommendations for depression
Recovery record, Rise up and Recover	Meal tracking for eating disorders
nOCD, Worry Watch	Identify trigger points and coping skills for OCD
UCSF PRIME, Schizophrenia Healthstory	Symptoms trackers for schizophrenia
PTSD Coach, Breath2Relax	Self assessment, positive self talk designed for PTSD
Headspace, Calm	Guided medication, mindfulness apps

FUTURE DIRECTION

Utilizing the availability of mobile devices and their passive data collections, health care providers would have a more comprehensive picture of patient's day to day functioning to assist in personalizing a more thorough treatment plan for the patient. Currently the most accurate form of monitoring called Ecological Momentary Assessment (EMA), also known as Experience Sampling Method (ESM). This system allows collection of real time information and assessment of behaviors, moods, thoughts, symptoms as well as daily experience in a patient's normal milieu. Some of the examples of assessment tools that would use the EMA system would be daily diary where patient would report their activities at the end of the day; signal dependent reporting where patient reports the symptoms or moods at random time in response to a text or alarm; and event dependent reporting is which the patient reports their mood or reaction to a challenging or distressing event that they have just recently experienced. Through this model, signal dependent and event dependent are most likely to be accurate since they are in vivo assessment. Through this method, the model would allow the physician to observe passively the symptoms over time rather than just a cross sectional self-report. This would allow the providers to see the variability of symptoms manifested in different social contexts.

EMA could incorporate daily assessment that would utilize the current style of apps which are the questionnaire style such as PHQ-2, PHQ-9 on a daily basis. This would be a more efficient assessment method for mood reporting. For psychotic disorder, a daily report of symptoms severity, mood, medication compliance would be able to alert care provider any deviation from the normal baseline. A study of 17 patients with schizophrenia utilized daily report, call logs and GPS data to predict the rate of relapse by analyzing how patients interacts with their smart phones. The conclusion was that the rate of behavioral anomalies was 71% higher within the 2 weeks prior to relapse. While this is a limited study with a small sample size, it demonstrated the potential of frequent passive monitoring for assessment and management of mental illness.

Currently, the new concept called Digital phenotyping is being incorporated into apps development. Digital phenotyping allows the mobile device to perform real time capture of a patient's clinical status. This may seem like a novel model, the traditional version had been utilized extensively in clinical care. Physicians often asked patient about sleep pattern, exercise level, appetite etc as a mean to measure their normal functioning baseline. With smart phones and accessories, it would be possible to capture patient's sleep pattern, activity level, basic vital signs passively rather than relying on the patients' recollection especially when visits are often monthly. Mobile devices are equipped with technologies that would allow capturing data passively through the use of sensor, accelerometer and GPS system.

DESIGNING THE IDEAL ASSESSMENT APP

When building an assessment, one has to conceptualize the level of data and engagement of not only its user but of the evaluator as well. In digital data, there are four types that can be collected through various means, this can be grouped into active data which requires user input and passive data:

1. Active reporting: daily surveys and self report questionnaires of patient's perceived symptoms
2. Active engagement: random scheduled tasks that require the user to actively engage in specific task to gather performance report. With touch screen, it would even be possible to see how patient performs a task, such as the number tracing task in MOCA, the device is sophisticated enough to measure the movements made on the screen.

3. Passive report: basic values such as sleep time, heart rates, activity levels can be measured through GPS and accelerometer
4. Passive activities: internet activities, social media activities. This can be utilized to detect certain key words for risk assessment.

These collected data can then be compiled and arranged as a report for not only the user but can be presented to the provider during follow up visits. These reports would assist in treatment modification. A hypothetical case would demonstrate what an ideal, all-inclusive assessment and monitoring app would be:

Mr A is a 30 year old male with history of major depressive disorder who came to an outpatient clinic to establish ongoing mental health care. During intake process, he would be given a tablet with general questions regarding his past psychiatric, medical and social history; he would also be required to write a basic message to the psychiatrist Dr B about any questions he might have. This would allow not only ease of information gathering but also the message that Mr A writes would be used to monitor how long it takes for him to complete the assessment, grammar, technical usage, corrections to establish an estimate of his mental status. As he waits for the psychiatrist, he can play a video game to evaluate his concentration, attention and psychomotor ability; the nurse can also enter patient's biographical data and vital signs into his chart.

Dr B would review the questionnaire with the patient and discuss any areas of concern as well as treatment options. This would establish Mr A's baseline of functioning. As a follow up, Dr B suggested that patient would download a client version of the same app used in the assessment to monitor his daily activities. This would allow data reporting patient's social and physical activities. The GPS would allow mapping of his area of activity, accelerometer would collect his level of physical activity, the internet activity can also be used to establish of his level of social involvement not only based on text, phone call activities but as well as the ones that were not answered. In addition, Mr A could have an option to get a smart watch that would allow routine monitoring of his vital signs, this can allow estimation of emotional state via skin conductance and cardiopulmonary activities; sleep can also be monitor through motion detection and heart rate. Once a week, Mr A would fill out a wellness survey; a compilation of his weekly data is displayed and compared to his baseline. A copy of the report can be sent to Dr B for evaluation. If there's a deviation from the norm, he started having less sleep, less physical activities, decline in social activities; together with his report, the psychiatrist would be able to determine if he needed to see the patient earlier for acute intervention or if any aspect of his treatment needed to be modified. The data collected routinely would be a means for measuring improvement or decline on a continuous basis.

LIMITATIONS

While it is possible and ideal to have such assessment tool, there are numerous factors that must be considered:

a Compliance: the importance of having such a comprehensive assessment tool such as this is the active participation of patients. While passive data can provide some suggestive estimate, the most useful information is the frequent utilization of reports. It would be meaningless if patient is unable or unwilling to participate.
b Security: the protection of personal data is the critical factor in developing such an app for frequent health monitoring. Extensive considerations, policies and laws have been developed to ensure that patient's private, personal health information is protected and available only to the essential parties. Having data on personal devices without the security measures like that of a hospital network is placing a patient's information at risk for cyber exploits.
c Privacy: while the majority of the world's population is comfortable to broadcast their thoughts, feelings, activities and locations into cyberspace, it is unknown as to how comfortable to

know that each of their movement is being compiled into a report for the purpose of psychiatric surveillance. This is perhaps the most controversial road block to overcome.

REFERENCES

Alvarez-Jimenez M, Alcazar-Corcoles M A, González-Blanch C, Bendall S, McGorry P D, Gleeson J F. Online, social media and mobile technologies for psychosis treatment: a systematic review on novel user-led interventions. *Schizophr. Res.* 2014; 156.

Arean P, Ly K., Andersson G. Mobile technology for mental health assessment. *Dialogues in clinical neuroscience,* June 2016; 18:2.

Barnett I., Torous J, Staples P. et al. Relapse prediction in schizophrenia through digital phenotyping: a pilot study. *Neuropsychopharmacology* 2018: 43.

Granholm, E, Ben-Zeev D., Link P., Bradshaw K., Holden J. Mobile assessment and treatment for schizophrenia (MATS): a pilot trial of an interactive text messaging intervention for medication adherence, socialization and auditory hallucinations. *Schizophrenia Bulletin,* May 2012; 28:3.

Hays Ryan, Torous J., Farrell H. Mobile apps and mental health: using technology to quantify real time clinical risk. *Current psychiatry,* June 2019; 18:6.

Marley J, Farooq S. Mobile telephone apps in mental health practice: uses, opportunities and challenges. *BJPsych Bulletin,* Dec 2015; 39:6.

Marshall J., Dunstan D., Bartik W. The digital psychiatrist: in search of evidence based apps for anxiety and depression. *Frontier in Psychiatry* 2019; 10:831.

Min Y H, Lee J W, Shin Y W, Jo M W, Sohn G, Lee J H, et al. Daily collection of self-reporting sleep disturbance data via a smartphone app in breast cancer patients receiving chemotherapy: a feasibility study. *J. Med. Internt. Res.* 2014; 16.

Palmier-Claus J., Rogers A., Ainsworth J., Matchin M. et al. Integrating mobile phone base assessment for psychosis into people's everyday lives and clinical care: a qualitative study. *BMC Psychiatry* 2013; 13:34.

Paris J., Phillips J. Making the DSM-5: concepts and Controversies. 2013.

Sedrati H., Nejjari C., Chaqsare S., Ghazal H. Mental and physical mobile health apps: review. *Procedia Computer Science*, 2016; 100.

Van Amerigen M., Turna J., Khalesi Z., Pullia K., Patterson B. There's an app for that! The current state of mobile applications for DSM-5 obsessive compulsive disorder, posttraumatic stress disorder, anxiety and mood disorder. *Depression and anxiety,* June 2017; 34:6.

Zhang M., Ho C., Ho R., Cheok C. Smartphone apps in mental healthcare: the state of the art and potential developments. *BJPsych. Advances* 2015; 21.

In: Innovations in Psychiatry
Editors: Souparno Mitra et al.
ISBN: 978-1-53619-365-7
© 2021 Nova Science Publishers, Inc.

Chapter 13

SOCIAL MEDIA AND ITS IMPACT ON MENTAL HEALTH

Noemi Edwards[*], *BA*
BronxCare Health System Department of Psychiatry
Icahn School of Medicine, Bronx, NY, US

ABSTRACT

In this chapter, we discuss the importance of something that has become ubiquitous with our life: social media. Whether it be Twitter, Instagram, Facebook or TikTok, social media is omnipotent and omnipresent. We discuss the impact of social media in our lives, in the mental health of patients and the ways and means that we can overcome the problems that come with social media use.

INTRODUCTION

Social media is a web-based platform that provides services to millions of people in the world. Social media was designed so that individuals

---

[*] Corresponding Author's Email: NEdwards@bronxcare.org.

around the world could share, create, and discuss almost anything. Social media has been seen to be a positive and an effective tool for organizations, businesses, politicians, public advocates, and government but has also been seen to negatively affect young teens and college students. Today there are millions of teens that own a social media account. While having opportunities to share and express opinions freely has been a benefit of social media, there are some challenges – particularly when information that is being shared is inappropriate, false, or inflammatory. This has become a global issue as some countries have found ways to censor social media, while others strongly enforce individuals to not have an existing account. While social media censorship is an advanced way to spread news, information, and pictures, it has lost its importance of being a tool that people used to connect with others, marketing, and promote businesses. It is now widely used to falsify information, cause depression in teens and students, and has been the source of riots and controversy. It has been a challenge for social media administrators to monitor what is being posted and for parents even more of a challenge to monitor teen's usage of social media at home.

THE RIGHT TO COMMUNICATE ON SOCIAL MEDIA

Social media censorship has been an ongoing global societal issue for some time now. While many believe social media censorship is a great idea, others find that it violates the First Amendment. Many users confuse the right to freedom of speech and expression with defamation or incitement (Heins, 2014), which is the cause of many debates on social media censorship. There are several countries including China that ban social media completely and find that it has been very successful (Pan, 2017). Entire continents such as Africa have tried to adopt this approach have been unsuccessful thus far. Social media censorship has proven to have many pros and cons. Recently, the impact of not censoring social media created a frenzy across a nation when individuals could not decipher real versus fake news.

MENTAL HEALTH AND SOCIAL MEDIA

The negative effects of social media also include implications towards mental health. In one study looking at Turkish adolescent students who were described as having an addiction to social media, they found an increased prevalence in depression in both high school students and college students. Depression is a major mental health issue and there are millions of youth that experience at least one period of depression in their adolescence (Kircaburun, 2016). "Nearly 75% of all teenagers between the ages of 13–17 report having an active Facebook account. Although adolescents view Facebook as an important tool in their social lives, some types of Facebook activity may predict increases in depression, loneliness, and a negative self-image" (Ehrenreich & Underwood, p. 228, 2016). Teens are overexposed to things that are posted on social media. A term coined "Facebook depression" usually occurs when individuals see profiles of others that maybe doing better than they are, traveling more, having what is perceived to be better relationships and a "better life." The implications to naïve adolescents who are unable to decipher reality from a perfect picture can be deadly.

Additionally, social media has been known to be the cause of riots and controversy, according to Baker, "new social media played a key role in organizing the recent riots with smart phones giving those with access to these technologies the power to network socially and to incite collective disorder" (Baker, 2012). Individuals are able to post messages and pictures in an instant. This does not give news spokesmen or women time to broadcast or write an article with actual facts. By the time an actual article is posted people all over the world would already have access which has led to devastating outcomes. Fuchs goes on to describe a riot in the UK in 2011, Blackberry Messenger and Twitter were the ignition to the fuel of the comments posted by dissenters and for this, the riots spread and the consequences were dire.

When looking at ways to reduce the global issues that social media causes one would be to have a stricter policy on who is able to use it and how it is used. A strict policy such as one similar to China would help keep unethical behavior under control. China's "government is not able to monitor all online content, so Internet companies in China are responsible for illegal content on their websites. The government publicly warned Weibo about inefficient censorship. To avoid being shut down by the government, these companies have hired censors to manually filter negative posts." This would eliminate all falsified and inappropriate behavior. In the article, protecting the innocence of youth: Moral sanctity values underlie censorship from young children it reviewed the definition of censorship, which is a form of protecting children from seeing immoral acts and keeping their purity. In a study that was conducted, it showed that "people who value moral sanctity tended also to value protecting young children from viewing immoral acts. Showing immoral acts to young children may violate ideals of moral sanctity, given that such acts involve tarnishing young children's purity and innocence" (Anderson & Masicampo, p. 14, 2017). In this case parents should be more involved and monitor what their children are doing on social media. Before any child is allowed to proceed with creating an account, a parent authority should be required to read a policy informing them of what their child may witness, and inform them that children more often become depressed after seeing social media posts by other friends and posters. Parents must sign off on this, that they were indeed notified of the possibilities of their child coming across unethical behavior. Parents can also put parental control on the tablets, phones and iPad. Currently, social media sites are being held accountable to do additional monitoring, but this is not consistent across all sites and not all sites remain accountable.

THE IMPACT OF SOCIAL MEDIA

Social media plays a role in every aspect of one's lives whether we have awareness or not. Social media is now used for job recruitment, sports, business, politics and health sector, it has even found widespread usage in public libraries. A recent study looked at the social media usage of the public library system and found that a staggering 61% of libraries have been using social media for 3 years or more, 30% post their information on social media daily, 25% of libraries have more than 5 individuals updating their social media pages, Facebook is the most popular social media channel, and 72% of libraries have no social media policy or plan in place. (Kumar & Agrawal, 2017).

The negative impact on the self-esteem of adolescents who use social media continues to rise. Study after study shows that social media does cause harm in young children and the recommendations for the government to take further steps to monitor content viewed by minors is on the rise.

Aside from the direct impact on mental health, social media through its anonymity has created an environment where its users' way of life had been slowly transformed and forced its way to be embedded intimately into people's lives. First and foremost, bullying has evolved into cyberbullying where anyone anywhere in the world can be affected. No longer will your bully have to wait until lunch hour, they can target you any time, any place, anywhere; all made possible by the extensive reach of social media. Additionally, a phenomenon known as FOMO (fear of missing out) has led to an increase in anxiety out of fear of missing out on the positive experience that others are having. People have become addicted with checking out their social media at times upwards of fifty to one hundred times per day to ensure they haven't missed out on anything; this leads to unhealthy and unsafe behaviors. Social media addiction may also create unrealistic expectation as well as negative self-image about one's own life and experiences.

Table 1. Mental Health conditions negatively impacted by social media

Mental Health Conditions	Social media's impact
Depression	Can worsen or exaccerbate a depressive episode
Anxiety	May increase anxiety in users
Cyberbullying	Creates more instances in bullying due to anonymity
Racial discrimination	Mass discrimination from different reaches of the world Based on online post
Fear of Missing Out	Creates anxiety and jealousy based on the experiences of others
Negative self image/ unrealistic expectation	Worsens self image by creating unhealthy and unrealistic models via numerous "influencers" promoting unhealthy habits

While it is easy to identify all of the potentially negative consequences and the negative impact of social media on society, it is also important to appreciate its' positive attributes and contributions to society at large. Foremost, social media has provided a platform where people can maintain a sense of community and connectedness with old friends and new. Users are able to form new connections based on old ones. This allows those who are anxious about engaging in social settings with others to be able to expand their network with the touch of a few buttons. There are support groups, social groups that help provide new relationships between those with common interests or are in need of support. Social media can also afford us the opportunity to share our life experience anonymously with less fear of being judged. This allows people to be more empathic and appreciative of others and learn from others' experiences.

SOCIAL MEDIA, WHAT TO DO?

Social media censorship clearly has its pros and cons. The financial implications of censorship to social media sites may in the long-term impact employment, financial solvability of social media companies as many users may not want to participate in a social community where they are not able to employ freedom of speech. While freedom of speech remains an integral part of our society, appreciating the devastating implications to adolescents who unsafely are exposed to this content has significant mental health consequences. In addition to depression, there is also social media addiction and sleep deprivation from the long hours of internet usage. While no one wants to feel like their rights are being taken away, there needs to be critical understanding of the short- and long-term consequences on minors.

In conclusion, social media is an advanced way to spread news, information, and pictures, and while originally was a tool used to inspire social connections, it is now connected to false content, increases in depression among youth and political controversy. I Ideally, social media should be a place where it is safe to log in, not having to worry that your or anyone's child will be affected.

REFERENCES

Anderson, R. A., & Masicampo, E. J. (2017). Protecting the innocence of youth: moral sanctity values underlie censorship from young children. *Personality and Social Psychology Bulletin*. 43(11), 1503–1518.

Baker, S. A. (2012). From the criminal crowd to the "mediated crowd:" the impact of social media on the 2011 English riots. *Safer Communities*, 11(1), 40. Retrieved from http://search.ebscohost.com.proxylibrary.ashford.edu/login.aspx?direct=true&db=edb&AN=70732652&site=eds-live&scope=site.

Behrmann, J. R. (2018). Speak your mind and ride the pine: examining the constitutionality of university-imposed social media bans on student-athletes. *The Jeffrey S. Moorad Sports Law Journal*, (1), 51.

Ehrenreich, S. E., & Underwood, M. K. (2016). Adolescents' internalizing symptoms as predictors of the content of their facebook communication and responses received from peers. *Translational Issues in Psychological Science,* 2(3), 227–237. http://doi.org/10.1037/tps0000077.

Fuchs, C. (2012). Social media, riots, and revolutions. (BEHIND THE NEWS) (Report). *Capital & Class*, Vol. 36, Issue 3, pp. 383 - 391. https://doi-org.proxy-library.ashford.edu/10.1177/03098168124 53613

Heins, M. (2014). *The brave new world of social media censorship: how "terms of service" abridge free speech.* Harvard Law Review Forum, 127(8), 325-330.

Kircaburun, K. (2016). Self-Esteem, daily internet use and social media addiction as predictors of depression among Turkish adolescents. *Journal of Education and Practice*, 7(24), 64–72.

Luqiu, L. R. (2017). The cost of humour: political satire on social media and censorship in China. *Global Media & Communication*, 13(2), 123. Retrieved from http://search.ebscohost.com.proxy-library.ashford.edu/login.aspx?direct=true&db=edb&AN=124458280&site=eds-live&scope=site.

Pan, J. (2017). How market dynamics of domestic and foreign social media firms shape strategies of internet censorship. *Problems of Post-Communism,* 64(3/4), 167–188.

Robb, A. 2017. Anatomy of a fake news scandal. *Rolling Stone.* Retreived from: https://www.rollingstone.com/politics/politics-news/anatomy-of-a-fake-news-scandal-125877/.

In: Innovations in Psychiatry
Editors: Souparno Mitra et al.

ISBN: 978-1-53619-365-7
© 2021 Nova Science Publishers, Inc.

Chapter 14

FUTURE DIRECTIONS

Shalini Dutta, MD and Souparno Mitra, MD*
BronxCare Health System, Department of Psychiatry,
Icahn School of Medicine, Bronx, NY, USA

ABSTRACT

In this chapter we discuss the road ahead in the development of new tools and assessments in Psychiatry. We discuss the utility of Artificial Intelligence, Face Mapping Softwares, Telepsychiatry and other modalities. Technology is always progressing and improving and our chapter will give insight into some directions that the field of psychiatry can head down.

INTRODUCTION

Psychiatry is a field in constant evolution with rapid changes having occurred over the last half century. No longer are people institutionalized

---

* Corresponding Author's Email: SMitra@bronxcare.org.

in inhumane conditions, chained and subjected to gross negligence. Instead, there is now a push to harness the maximum capacity of technology and internet access to care for our patients in the most modern ways. This push is further bolstered by the current state of the world in this ongoing pandemic. Fields such as telehealth and an increasing number of applications geared towards the psychiatric population have been changing the landscape of psychiatric interactions between physicians and their patients.

However, a number of barriers exist to implementation of these technologies on both the patient and clinician side. The main areas of concern include compliance, security and privacy of the data exchanged. Users need to acquire technological devices, have proper network connectivity, and be a motivated participant. Clinicians need to be able to incorporate these new technologies into their daily work flow in a standardized manner. Future research development must occur to make sure such technologies are optimized and implemented in ways that will encourage compliance keeping patient's engaged in their own mental health care.

Future Directions in Different Realms

We review some of the possible advances that may increase the technological prowess in evaluation and management of psychiatric patients.

(a) Artificial intelligence and the future of psychiatry: Qualitative findings from a global physician survey.

A web-based survey of 791 psychiatrists from 22 counties took place in Spring 2019. The survey measured opinions about the likelihood future technology would replace physicians in performing ten key psychiatric tasks. Three open ended questions were also asked and analyzed. Comments were divided into 4 categories relating to the impact of future technology on patient- psychiatrist interactions, quality of patient medical care, profession of psychiatry and health systems.

Varied views pertaining to the influence of future technology on the status of the profession were elicited ranging from the opinion that psychiatrists would be completely replaced by artificial intelligence to the thinking that technology would have no effect on psychiatric services. The pervasive view shared by participants was that "man and machine" would work together in diagnosing and treatment decisions. Many survey responses suggested that AI would aid physician roles without ever fully taking over.

Many participants felt that diagnostic and clinical decisions would always be fulfilled by humans and that too much dependence on technology might drive medical error. There was also consideration given to the lack of empathy that may be expressed through technology. On a happier note, many participants felt technology would be more equitable and decrease human bias that may occur. There was an optimism that technology would take over more administrative duties. Some respondents felt that technology would improve access to psychiatric care, reduce costs and increase efficiency.

(b) ADHD Apps

Patients with ADHD are known to be forgetful and easy distractible and this affects their academic achievements if the symptoms are not addressed in a timely manner. However, they excel at playing video games due to various stimuli and reward systems involved in gaming. There are a number of technological applications used by millions of teachers, students and parents to aid in daily activities. Examples include "Class Dojo" a collaboration between teachers and parents on refining behavior, class participation and positive feedback from teachers. "Photomath" which helps children with ADHD by tutoring them and guiding then step wise to arrive at a solution. "Grade proof" checks spelling grammar and formatting errors for children with ADHD who are particularly prone to dyslexia and dysgraphia. Changes in social functioning, societal expectation coupled with increased access to internet and mobile devices are offering up unique ways for parents to engage their children in daily activities as well as monitor symptoms. These ADHD focused applications geared towards both caregiver and children warrants further exploration.

(c) Apps for anxiety

Similar to finding the right therapist, mental health applications need to be the right fit. There is currently immense competition among these applications in the online free market space which will encourage further development and improvement of app features. Applications for anxiety which assist with mindfulness and meditation are a dime a dozen. Customary free trial periods and features allow potential subscribers to make a well-informed choice from the comfort of their own home. This is certainly a golden period in terms of mental health awareness and technological development with only better things to come in the future.

We do need well designed randomized clinical trials to adequately check the efficacy of these apps.

(d) Psychological Testing Tools

Tools such as Ecological Momentary Assessment which is also known as Experience Sampling Method and Digital Phenotyping allow for real time assessments of a patient's daily life. Physicians can use such technologies to learn about their patients behavior in a multitude of ways in order to gain information. There is a great scope of developing this treatment and assessment modality via more user-friendly interfaces, applications which are more accessible to the patients and developing more and more assessment tools which are rooted in evidence.

(e) CBT

In this ongoing pandemic it is necessary to expand technology such as telemedicine to provide optimized patient care. The use of internet and computers to allow patients to engage in evidence-based modalities such as CBT is vital. Offering CBT in this manner breaks geographic boundaries (ensuring access to those that live in remote rural areas), provides a means of access for those that might not normally engage due to shame or fear of stigma, allows easy access from anywhere at any time, is cost and time efficient and enhances overall health literacy and high user acceptability. End user adoption of telehealth is challenged by the need to integrate such services into clinical practice work flow.

Further, adoption required cultural and behavioral changed for use and reliance on telehealth technologies. From a patient perspective, usability of these technologies is hampered by the lack of technology integration, interoperability and standardization. The key is putting the "person" in personalized medicine.

There is great scope of automated delivery of basic CBT training to meet the gaps in care. However, this requires a greater synthesis between the medical and technical arms of medical innovation to come up with ideas for these techniques.

(f) EMA

Ecological momentary assessment has been shown to be beneficial for real time assessment for disorders such as anxiety and substance use. Further research is need focusing on appropriate frequency and duration of EMA as well as the content of the assessments. Further study may improve compliance as well as lead to more effective and user friendly therapeutic results. The development of structured, protocolized administration frequency of EMA and more user-friendly interfaces may enable this technique to be more popular.

There is great scope for development of EMA as stated by Schuller et al., who found that many EMIs are limited in the treatment of depression and anxiety. The limitations are in the form of the need for the user to initiate the assessment and the interventions may often be clunky. There is scope for developing more integrative and personalized EMIs.

EMIs may be developed to detect the mental state of patients through passive sensors. Some studies have shown the initial data that passive sensing may be possible. The EMIs of the future may not need to ask people what they are feeling but rather tell them of the basis of passively collected data. EMIs could also be developed to provide personalized interventions for patents. This has been made possible by peer networks which provide content on demand. Advances in natural language and machine learning may automate the process.

Further, to enable greater accuracy of EMAs, longer duration studies should be run for EMAs being used for ambulatory physiological measurements.In terms of research there is a need to develop methodological guidelines similar to that being done for lab based measurements.

However, there is a great need to balance the needs of the patient with the needs of the provider as this innovation often needs motivation from patients.

Conclusion

This book describes some of the technological innovations that have occurred in psychiatry till today and also looks into the possibilities for the future.

With the advent of artificial intelligence and machine learbing, there is great scope for an objective assessment and also the opportunities to deliver individualized treatment for patients. Medical innovation is in an exciting times and these tools can increase the access to mental health care and serve as the crucial resource that much of society needs.

These are exciting times and there is great hope in the future that lies ahead.

REFERENCES

Blease, C., Locher, C., Leon-Carlyle, M., & Doraiswamy, M. (2020). Artificial intelligence and the future of psychiatry: Qualitative findings from a global physician survey. *Digital health*, 6, 2055207620968355. https://doi.org/10.1177/2055207620968355.

Schueller, S. M., Aguilera, A., & Mohr, D. C. (2017). Ecological momentary interventions for depression and anxiety. *Depression and anxiety*, 34(6), 540–545. https://doi.org/10.1002/da.22649.

ABOUT THE EDITORS

Souparno Mitra
Resident Psychiatry
Bronxcare Health System, Icahn School of Medicine at Mount Sinsai

Dr Souparno Mitra is a Psychiatry Resident at Bronxcare Health Systems. Prior to his residency, he worked as a primary care provider in India. He has published close to 10 papers and has given talks to national conferences. He was also awarded the AAAP Travel Award and the Research Colloquium Early Career Track Scholarship at the APA. He is extremely interested in addiction research and is also the Research Co-ordinator for the Bronxcare Psychiatry Research Lab.

Urmi Chaudhuri
PhD Student
Isenberg School of Management, University of Massachusettes, Amherst

Urmi Chaudhuri is a PhD Student in Strategic Management at the Isenberg School of Management at University of Massachusetts in Amherst. Prior to starting her PhD, she has also completed her Masters in Human Resources Management from Rutgers University. She is also an established Corporate Lawyer with 7 years of experience in India. She is interested in research in Technological innovations and Employee Ownership

Panagiota Korenis
Program Director and Vice Chair of Education
Icahn School of Medicine at Mount Sinai and Albert Einstein College of Medicine

Dr. Panagiota Korenis is Vice Chair and Residency Director for the Department of Psychiatry at Bronx Care Health System in New York. She is Associate Professor at Albert Einstein College of Medicine and is actively engaged in teaching psychiatry residents and medical students alike. Dr. Korenis has published and presented her work regionally, nationally and internationally. She has been recognized as an outstanding faculty mentor by the New York State Psychiatric Association.

INDEX

A

abuse, 77, 78, 80, 82
access, ix, x, 6, 7, 8, 9, 12, 14, 15, 17, 18, 19, 28, 29, 44, 45, 51, 53, 60, 61, 64, 68, 72, 73, 74, 75, 78, 81, 82, 91, 101, 132, 133, 134, 137, 139, 151, 158, 159, 161, 162
accessibility, x, 25, 44, 45, 82, 137, 140
ACT, 74
addiction, vii, 11, 17, 20, 79, 128, 130, 131, 132, 133, 134, 135, 142, 151, 153, 155, 156, 165
addiction counselling, 130
adolescents, 8, 14, 15, 49, 91, 95, 104, 106, 122, 124, 151, 153, 155, 156
adulthood, ix, 115, 118, 121
adults, 8, 14, 22, 30, 44, 50, 56, 60, 62, 104, 105, 119, 124
advancement, x, 137, 139, 140
advocacy, 2, 31, 112
age, ix, 6, 9, 14, 15, 16, 22, 27, 30, 48, 86, 101, 103, 109, 116, 121, 128, 129
alcohol use, 128, 131, 133, 139

American Board of Psychiatry and Neurology, 5
American Psychiatric Association, 2, 113, 116, 123, 138
antidepressant, 5, 42, 87
anxiety, v, viii, 4, 14, 21, 22, 23, 24, 25, 26, 28, 29, 30, 31, 34, 43, 44, 46, 47, 48, 49, 51, 55, 56, 57, 64, 86, 87, 89, 90, 93, 94, 96, 97, 98, 99, 100, 104, 110, 111, 113, 118, 123, 129, 130, 139, 141, 142, 147, 148, 153, 154, 160, 161, 163
Anxiety, 24, 30, 48, 90, 104, 113
anxiety disorder, 14, 22, 24
anxiety disorder(s), viii, 14, 21, 22, 23, 24, 30, 44, 48, 86, 90, 104, 110, 113, 118, 139
anxiety disorders in children, 104
AOT, 74
appointments, 12, 86, 93
apps for ADHD, 121
artificial intelligence, 7, 68, 158, 159, 162, 163
assertive community treatment, 3
assessment, vii, 1, 7, 8, 14, 19, 25, 50, 52, 55, 56, 64, 65, 86, 87, 89, 90, 91, 94, 97, 98, 99, 100, 112, 124, 133, 138, 140,

141, 142, 143, 144, 145, 146, 147, 148, 160, 161, 162
assessment tools, 89, 98, 112, 138, 140, 141, 143, 160
assisted outpatient treatment, 2
asylum, 2, 18, 20
asylums, vii, 1, 2, 9
Attention Deficit Hyperactivity Disorder (ADHD), vi, ix, 15, 90, 102, 115, 116, 117, 118, 119, 120, 121, 122, 123, 124, 159
awareness, 78, 153, 160

B

barriers, 5, 8, 12, 61, 132, 158
base, 7, 50, 66, 121, 133, 148
behavior therapy, 47, 55, 132
behaviors, 22, 23, 61, 65, 67, 68, 93, 100, 106, 117, 130, 142, 143, 153
benefits, vii, 11, 12, 17, 47, 49, 51, 53, 64, 66, 77, 82, 92, 99
BHCC, 82
bias, 46, 55, 88, 92, 98, 159
binge eating disorder, 52, 60, 63, 66, 67, 69, 96
binge-eating disorder (BED), 51, 53
bipolar disorder in children, 103
Boylan Act, 73
brain, 5, 36, 117, 119, 128, 131
breathing, 28, 73, 107
bulimia, 51, 52, 58, 61, 63
bulimia nervosa, 51, 52, 58, 63

C

California Triplicate Prescription Program, 73
caregivers, ix, 93, 101, 105, 122
CBT, 44
CBTI, 50, 51
c-CBT, v, viii, 43, 44, 45, 46, 47, 48, 49, 50, 51
censorship, 150, 152, 155, 156
challenges, vii, viii, 7, 8, 11, 15, 17, 18, 22, 35, 43, 69, 147, 150
childhood, ix, 34, 103, 115, 116, 124
children, ix, 8, 14, 15, 86, 95, 101, 102, 103, 104, 105, 106, 107, 109, 119, 122, 124, 152, 153, 155, 159
China, 150, 152, 156
class dojo, 121, 159
classification, 117, 133, 138
clients, 27, 29, 75
cocaine, 86, 87, 98, 129, 132, 133
cognition, 8, 64, 86, 92, 93
cognitive behavioral therapy (CBT), viii, 8, 22, 26, 30, 43, 44, 45, 46, 47, 48, 49, 50, 51, 53, 54, 55, 56, 57, 61, 63, 65, 66, 67, 119, 130, 131, 134, 142, 160, 161
cognitive behavioral therapy for insomnia (CBTI), 50
collaboration, 12, 17, 122, 141, 159
commercial, 3, 47, 61
communication, 6, 27, 44, 67, 83, 102, 140, 142, 156
community/communities, viii, 8, 16, 17, 26, 28, 53, 59, 61, 79, 99, 128, 132, 133, 154, 155
Community Mental Health Act, 2
compliance, 12, 42, 52, 66, 99, 158, 161
computer, ix, 8, 9, 44, 45, 56, 60, 64, 101
computerized- Cognitive Behavioral Therapy (c-CBT), 44
connectivity, 99, 117, 158
consumers, 4, 65, 67, 141
contingency, 97, 98, 132
control group, 46, 51, 65
controlled substances, 72, 77, 78, 79
conversion disorder (functional neurological symptom disorder) in children, 106

correctional facilities, 18
cost, 17, 25, 27, 45, 46, 47, 53, 55, 61, 65, 79, 132, 134, 156, 161
cycles, vii, 1, 4

D

database, ix, 71, 73, 74, 76, 77, 78, 142
day one, 38
DBT, 23
deficit, ix, 96, 115, 121, 123, 124
depression, viii, 15, 16, 30, 43, 44, 45, 46, 47, 48, 49, 50, 54, 55, 56, 57, 91, 93, 94, 100, 104, 129, 130, 139, 141, 142, 147, 150, 151, 155, 156, 161, 163
depressive symptoms, 8, 34, 49, 56, 104, 109, 110
diagnostic criteria, x, 127, 138
dialectical behavioral therapy, 23, 28
Diarium, 38
diffusion phase, 3, 4
digital phenotyping, 8, 144, 147, 160
disorder, ix, 17, 22, 23, 49, 50, 51, 53, 60, 61, 63, 64, 65, 66, 67, 68, 96, 103, 106, 111, 115, 116, 118, 120, 121, 123, 124, 128, 129, 130, 134, 138, 139, 140, 143, 148, 151
disruptive, impulsive-control and conduct disorders, 108
dissociative disorders in children, 105
distress, 23, 34, 139
Dorothea Dix, 2
dream journal, 36
drugs, 2, 87, 128, 129, 131, 134

E

early warning signs questionnaire, 93
eating disorder(s) (ED), viii, 30, 43, 44, 51, 52, 53, 57, 58, 59, 60, 61, 62, 63, 64, 65, 66, 67, 68, 69, 73, 81, 94, 95, 96, 106, 142
eating disorders, viii, 30, 43, 44, 51, 57, 58, 59, 60, 61, 62, 63, 64, 65, 66, 67, 68, 94, 95, 142
ecological momentary assessment, vi, ix, 63, 66, 85, 86, 87, 90, 92, 94, 95, 96, 99, 100, 143, 160, 161
education, 12, 69, 82, 119, 129, 132, 140, 142
EKG, 90, 96, 97
elimination disorders in children, 107
emergency, 12, 15, 74, 75, 78, 80, 83
Emil Kraeplin, 2
emotion, 8, 13, 23
England, 54, 55, 56
environment, 12, 23, 24, 45, 88, 94, 153
e-therapy, 62, 89, 90
Eugene Beuler, 2
evidence, vii, viii, 7, 8, 11, 14, 22, 25, 30, 43, 44, 46, 48, 49, 50, 51, 53, 60, 61, 62, 64, 65, 68, 121, 122, 124, 132, 133, 134, 147, 160, 161
evolution, 21, 140, 157
exercise(s), 2, 29, 41, 64, 65, 67, 89, 107, 142, 144
expertise, 18, 61, 68
exposure, 12, 24, 75

F

Facebook, x, 149, 151, 153
families, 16, 121, 128, 131
FDA, 8, 119, 121, 122
fear, 53, 79, 80, 104, 132, 153, 154, 161
fear of missing out, 153, 154
feelings, viii, 14, 33, 34, 42, 106, 146
financial, 25, 87, 109, 129, 155
fitness, 28, 65, 67
fluid vulnerability report, 92
FOCUS, 93, 141

freedom, 67, 150, 155
freedom of speech, 150, 155
Freud, 2, 5, 138
future directions, vi, 8, 81, 94, 95, 100, 157, 158

G

gender dysphoria, 108
Generalized Anxiety Disorder, 86, 104, 110
goal planning journals, 35
Google, 7, 42, 132, 133
GPS, 143, 144, 145
gratitude journaling, 35
group therapy, 5, 12, 24
guardian, ix, 15, 101
guidelines, 56, 58, 142, 162

H

hallucinations, 97, 103, 147
harm reduction, 134
HARP status, 74
health, viii, x, 2, 6, 7, 8, 12, 15, 16, 17, 18, 19, 21, 22, 25, 26, 27, 28, 29, 30, 34, 39, 43, 44, 47, 51, 53, 58, 60, 61, 62, 63, 65, 68, 69, 72, 73, 75, 81, 106, 112, 127, 131, 132, 133, 139, 141, 142, 143, 146, 148, 151, 153, 159, 160, 161, 163
health care, 2, 8, 12, 16, 25, 44, 73, 132, 140, 141, 142, 143
health condition, 15, 16, 44
health information, 68, 72, 146
health services, viii, 28, 43, 47
heart rate, 63, 145, 146
heroin, 80, 129, 132
high school, 86, 129, 151
HIPAA, 6, 72, 81, 89

history, vii, ix, 1, 39, 52, 72, 73, 75, 76, 77, 78, 79, 80, 81, 86, 92, 115, 118, 123, 124, 129, 138, 145
human, 8, 18, 21, 22, 123, 159
hyperactivity, ix, 96, 102, 109, 115, 116, 121, 123, 124

I

ideal(s), 145, 146, 152
Illness Anxiety Disorder, 106
image(s), 12, 38, 154
improvements, 52, 78, 81, 82
impulsivity, ix, 115, 116
inattention, ix, 102, 109, 115, 118
individuals, 3, 16, 19, 25, 26, 44, 45, 50, 51, 52, 53, 60, 61, 66, 67, 92, 109, 110, 117, 128, 131, 132, 133, 134, 149, 151, 153
industry, 9, 28, 62
innovation phase, 3
insomnia, viii, 43, 44, 50, 51, 56
institutionalized, 2, 157
integration, 12, 53, 95, 134, 161
intelligence, 7, 68, 118, 158, 159, 162, 163
intervention, ix, 44, 46, 47, 48, 56, 61, 63, 68, 75, 78, 82, 85, 93, 99, 130, 131, 142, 146, 147
inventions, x, 127, 132
issues, viii, 7, 14, 15, 25, 27, 43, 45, 49, 90, 95, 96, 152

L

laws, 72, 83, 146
lead, 14, 61, 66, 79, 99, 130, 161
learning, viii, 28, 43, 68, 94, 103, 130, 162
list of screening tools, 109

M

machine learning, 7, 68, 94, 162
majority, 16, 25, 26, 27, 37, 94, 133, 134, 146
management, 12, 16, 17, 50, 56, 67, 87, 93, 98, 132, 142, 144, 158
manic, 103, 104, 138
Massachusetts General Hospital, 5, 139, 140
measurement(s), 8, 63, 95, 97, 162
media, x, 7, 37, 38, 121, 145, 147, 149, 150, 151, 152, 153, 154, 155, 156
Medicaid, 27, 72, 74, 76, 134
Medicaid ID, 74
medical, 12, 16, 17, 19, 27, 52, 72, 73, 77, 78, 80, 106, 128, 139, 140, 141, 142, 145, 159, 161, 166
medication, 2, 14, 16, 75, 79, 80, 87, 88, 93, 119, 128, 142, 143, 147
medication assisted treatment, 17, 130
medication compliance, 88, 93, 142, 143
medications for ADHD, 120
medicine, 20, 53, 54, 56, 161
memory, vii, 1, 86, 88, 117
mental disorder, x, 5, 51, 63, 123, 124, 135, 137, 138, 140
mental health, viii, ix, x, 2, 3, 6, 7, 8, 9, 12, 15, 16, 18, 20, 25, 26, 27, 28, 29, 30, 33, 43, 46, 50, 51, 56, 57, 60, 61, 62, 64, 65, 67, 69, 86, 112, 115, 116, 128, 138, 140, 141, 142, 145, 147, 148, 149, 151, 153, 155, 158, 160, 162
mental health monitoring, 139
mental illness, viii, ix, 1, 2, 5, 8, 17, 18, 21, 22, 25, 44, 101, 102, 135, 138, 144
messages, 61, 64, 92, 96, 151
meta-analysis, 19, 45, 49, 57, 94
methodology, ix, 85, 88
misuse, 72, 77, 79, 107
mobile apps, viii, x, 59, 61, 65, 67, 96, 127, 132, 141, 147
mobile device, viii, 43, 60, 64, 67, 122, 140, 143, 144, 160
mobile EKG and EEGs, 90
mobile phone, x, 36, 44, 60, 96, 127, 132, 148
models, 4, 9, 154
mood disorder, 118, 138, 148
motivation, 23, 41, 65, 99, 162
motivational interviewing, 28, 130
music, 2, 29, 38

N

National Health Service (NHS), 6, 7, 51, 61
National Health Service (NHS)
NCS, 119, 124, 125
Nebraska Psychiatric Institute, 5
neurobiology of ADHD, 116
neurodevelopment disorders, 102
New York State Office of Mental Health, 72, 75
NHS, 6, 7, 51, 61
NSSI, 91

O

obsessive compulsive and related disorder, 105
OCD, 23, 111, 139, 142
opioid use, 17, 80, 133
opioids, 72, 77, 79, 82, 84, 134
opportunities, 6, 12, 60, 147, 150, 162
outpatient, 50, 86, 87, 128, 130, 145

P

pain, 42, 44, 72, 78, 79, 82, 95
panic disorder, 44, 97, 139
parents, ix, 16, 101, 118, 119, 121, 122, 129, 150, 152, 159

participants, 16, 24, 47, 52, 53, 66, 67, 91, 95, 96, 159
password, 38, 39, 133
patient care, 9, 72, 75, 160
PDMP, v, ix, 71, 72, 73, 77, 78, 79, 80, 81, 82
peer support, 8, 133, 134
personal digital assistants, 90
pharmacotherapy for anxiety disorder, 24
physicians, 73, 78, 79, 80, 116, 158
platform, 34, 38, 68, 133, 149, 154
playing, 29, 38, 117, 121, 159
policy, 19, 72, 80, 112, 135, 152, 153
population, viii, 15, 16, 18, 22, 25, 27, 37, 43, 50, 58, 60, 66, 69, 76, 119, 138, 146, 158
post-traumatic stress disorder, viii, 43, 44
prescription drug monitoring programs, 72, 83, 84
prevention, 128, 131, 134, 139, 142
principles, viii, 59, 63, 86, 88, 130
protection, 38, 133, 146
psychiatric assessment, 19, 138
psychiatrist, 12, 15, 26, 27, 87, 140, 145, 146, 147, 159
psychiatry, vii, x, 1, 2, 4, 5, 9, 11, 15, 16, 19, 30, 54, 55, 81, 100, 125, 138, 140, 147, 157, 158, 159, 162, 163, 166
psychology, 40, 100, 123
psychology online, 6
psychopathology, 52, 53, 64, 67
psychophysiological applications, 96, 100
psychosis, 8, 44, 92, 147, 148
psychotherapy, 16, 44, 54, 119
PSYCKES, v, ix, 71, 72, 73, 74, 75, 76, 77, 81, 82, 83
PTSD, viii, 8, 15, 22, 23, 43, 97, 111, 139, 141, 142

Q

quality of life, 49, 52, 117

R

rating scale, 25, 26, 131, 132, 133, 138
real time, 64, 66, 87, 91, 98, 99, 121, 143, 144, 147, 160, 161
reality, 68, 117, 129, 151
recall, 88, 95, 98, 105, 121, 140
recommendations, 15, 42, 49, 142, 153
recovery, x, 66, 81, 127, 132, 133
reflective journaling, 34
relaxation, 25, 28, 94
reliability, 4, 7, 140
researchers, 7, 9, 62, 67, 88
resilience, xi, 22, 30, 89
resources, ix, 6, 8, 26, 47, 74, 98, 101, 132, 133, 134, 139
response, 21, 64, 75, 86, 88, 93, 96, 98, 105, 119, 132, 143
risk, 50, 67, 68, 72, 78, 82, 90, 92, 102, 109, 118, 128, 130, 134, 139, 145, 146, 147
risk factors, 92, 128, 130
Rosemary Kennedy, 2
rural areas, 12, 14, 26, 51, 161

S

safety, 14, 45, 46, 49, 53, 80, 92, 142
schizophrenia, 2, 103, 118, 142, 143, 147
schizophrenia in childhood, 103
school, 15, 16, 28, 95, 96, 104, 118, 119, 121, 124, 129
science, 7, 9, 134
scope, 9, 99, 155, 156, 160, 161, 162
security, 14, 74, 80, 91, 108, 146, 158
self-monitoring, 67, 68, 94
self-monitoring program, 61

sensor(s), 7, 8, 94, 97, 144, 162
services, 2, 5, 6, 12, 16, 17, 18, 30, 45, 47, 49, 53, 61, 63, 68, 74, 76, 86, 99, 132, 133, 134, 135, 139, 149, 159, 161
shame, 53, 60, 161
signs, 80, 88, 93, 106, 140, 144, 145
skin, 97, 105, 145
sleep-wake disorders in children, 107
smart phone, x, 30, 60, 66, 67, 68, 137, 139, 143, 144, 151
SMS, 61, 93, 132
social anxiety, 44, 46, 51
social media, x, 7, 37, 145, 147, 149, 150, 151, 152, 153, 154, 155, 156
society, 3, 21, 60, 154, 155, 162
solution, 19, 90, 122, 159
somatic symptom disorder, 106
speech, 38, 73, 102, 103, 150, 155, 156
spelling, 36, 122, 159
standardization, 51, 53, 161
state, 26, 31, 72, 73, 77, 82, 94, 104, 148, 158
states, 16, 17, 27, 29, 77, 82, 97, 105, 128
stigma, 8, 9, 16, 53, 64, 132, 161
stress, viii, 22, 43, 94
stressors, 87, 89, 90, 105
substance abuse, 23, 44, 78, 80, 81
substance use, x, 6, 15, 18, 23, 74, 78, 80, 92, 95, 96, 97, 98, 99, 118, 120, 127, 128, 129, 130, 132, 133, 134, 139, 161
substance use disorder(s), x, 96, 127, 128, 132, 133, 134
substance-related and addictive disorders, 109
substitution phase, 3, 4
suicide, 25, 90, 91, 129, 139
symptoms, 48, 49, 51, 52, 64, 65, 67, 80, 87, 90, 92, 94, 95, 97, 98, 103, 104, 105, 106, 108, 109, 116, 122, 138, 139, 140, 141, 143, 144, 156, 159
syndication phase, 3

T

target, 49, 94, 132, 153
teachers, 102, 118, 119, 121, 122, 159
techniques, 8, 28, 63, 89, 130, 161
technological advancement, 4, 5, 15
technological advances, 4, 44, 66, 68
Technological Life Cycles (TLC), 3
technology/technologies, vii, x, 1, 3, 4, 6, 7, 8, 12, 14, 29, 44, 45, 52, 53, 55, 56, 57, 58, 61, 63, 66, 68, 72, 93, 95, 99, 100, 121, 122, 132, 137, 139, 144, 147, 151, 157, 158, 159, 160, 161
telehealth, 19, 28, 53, 58, 158, 161
telemedicine, 12, 14, 15, 16, 19, 58, 160
telephone, 47, 56, 147
telepsychiatry, v, vii, x, 1, 4, 5, 8, 11, 12, 13, 14, 15, 16, 17, 18, 19, 20, 31, 157
testing, 4, 5, 74, 92, 141
therapist, 23, 44, 45, 49, 51, 52, 87, 98, 160
therapy, viii, 4, 6, 12, 14, 23, 25, 27, 28, 29, 30, 43, 45, 47, 49, 50, 51, 52, 54, 55, 56, 57, 58, 59, 60, 62, 63, 65, 87, 89, 90, 94, 98, 119, 130, 131, 142
thoughts, viii, 22, 33, 34, 35, 36, 38, 41, 92, 106, 143, 146
training, 20, 25, 80, 140, 161
trauma and stressor related disorders in children, 105
treatment, vii, viii, ix, 1, 2, 6, 8, 14, 15, 17, 18, 22, 34, 42, 43, 44, 45, 46, 47, 48, 49, 50, 51, 52, 53, 54, 55, 58, 59, 60, 61, 63, 64, 65, 66, 69, 72, 74, 76, 77, 78, 80, 81, 87, 88, 89, 92, 93, 94, 95, 97, 98, 115, 119, 128, 130, 131, 132, 133, 134, 135, 138, 140, 141, 142, 143, 145, 147, 159, 160, 161, 162
treatment of ADHD, 119
trial, 30, 45, 47, 51, 54, 55, 56, 58, 65, 147, 160
triggers, 87, 89, 97, 98, 132

twelve step facilitation, 131

U

United States (USA), viii, 5, 15, 16, 18, 21, 22, 30, 31, 72, 73, 78, 80, 83, 123, 129, 135, 157

V

videos, 12, 28, 38, 39
virtual reality, 7, 68

W

Washington, 20, 31, 99, 135
web, 28, 62, 81, 83, 122, 149, 158
web-based platform, 149
well-being, 27, 34, 131
wellness, viii, 43, 146
worry, 79, 104, 155

X

Xenzone, 6